WELLNESS LOADING

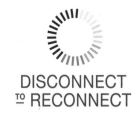

DISCONNECT ᵀᴼ RECONNECT

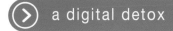
a digital detox

ANDI LEW

RICH
ALS

First published in Australia in 2016 by Heart to Heart Publishing

Postal: 20 Ormond Rd, Elwood, VIC, 3184
Tel: 0415 752 351
Fax: 03 9531 3131
Email: andi_lew@yahoo.com
Website: www.andilew.com

A Cataloguing-in-Publication entry is available from the National Library of Australia.

ISBN: 978-0-9873504-7-3 (pbk.)
ISBN: 978-0-9873504-8-0 (eBook)

Cover photography by Fernanda Ramos FR Group
Cover layout and design by Vanessa Russell (www.raspberrycreative.com.au)
Edited by iinspire media
Printed by BPA Printing

slide to open

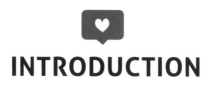

INTRODUCTION

Are you too attached to your phone?
I am the first to admit that I am. I *am* addicted.

But how do we stop something that has - in all fairness - improved our lives by so much? Because that's really the bottom line. We have more access to so much more information and networks. We have been able to connect with people we wouldn't normally have been able to reach. On the flip side, we often don't notice the people or moments right there in front of us because we are all too busy looking down ... not up!

In the lead up to writing this book, everyone I spoke to admitted they were in need of a digital detox. After many conversations, I soon I realised there wasn't one person that didn't want some 'time out' from their phone but they didn't know how.

So many people said to me "Hand over your book now! I need it in my life!" It was said in jest, but there's an element of truth in every joke. That's why jokes are funny. I also noticed a hint of desperation in this statement because we know we have to eventually get a handle on our digital addiction. But 'how' is the hardest part.

That is why I just had to write this book! I felt compelled to create something to help you use your technology a little less. I believe the key is to not stop using our devices altogether, but rather add a little balance to our lives.

Let me draw an analogy: so many of us crave ice-cream but we know it's bad for us as it's full of sugar. Too much and we suffer. Too little and we're always thinking about it! We need to find a way to moderate our intake. The same can be said for our digital consumption. By having ice-cream and our 'device' as a 'sometimes treat' means that when we choose to have it (or use it), it is all the more meaningful, enjoyable and even purposeful.

But how hard is this when you use technology for work and you have a sedentary job? I believe that even then, there are still ways of creating balance and I hope to show you these in this book. You will see that when in balance, your use of technology through consciously chosen periods of time will enhance your enjoyment and the tech's usefulness.

Conversely, when you decide to 'turn off tech', you just as consciously decide to really tune out. You create a 'knowing' that you will be able to go back to your device again with proper commitment to that task.

> And that's because you **chose** to reconnect when you chose to disconnect.

In our fast paced modern world, we are doing more but can often achieve less or even 'be' less. Have you ever found yourself going to respond to a message, only to get caught up scrolling through photos of your friend's mum's boyfriend's colleague's cat and thought, "How on earth did I get on here?" It can all become a little mindless. At times, we don't even realise because our phones can get us so side-tracked.

It's human nature to get side-tracked and easily distracted. Look at the ancient story of Adam and Eve. A prime case of obvious distraction! Ok, maybe not such a good example but the point is; we all do it. It doesn't help that as a society, everything seems faster - our ads are quicker, messages shorter and acronyms suffice for words. LOL, ROTFL, DVD, FOMO, CEO, do I need to go on? We have created a demand for 'quick'.

It's ok to be distracted when we want to disconnect and do something mindless, especially if we have had a stressful day. But we must be aware of not getting trapped in the fruitlessness of it all, especially when it becomes something we do on a regular basis. We used to have set times to choose to be mindless and watch an entertaining movie or read a book. We were able to be disconnected in a wonderful way, maybe once a week. Now, as we have so much access, our 'downtime' is no longer planned or scheduled, but rather just anytime and all day, every day!

As cliché as it sounds, it really is all about balance. You often hear people saying, don't give up the wine, the chocolate, or any other indulgence. Rather "have it in moderation", which is just another word for 'balance'. After all, trying to go 'cold turkey' may leave you wanting it even more initially. What you resist, persists.

I'm not advocating a total cessation of using your 'tech'. But why can't we find a healthier substitute for a planned period of time? Won't this reconnection to our 'real life' world be most beneficial?

As a certified Food, Lifestyle and Wellness Coach, I will show you how that is all possible through the pages of *Wellness Loading: Disconnect to Reconnect*. You will learn about what I call

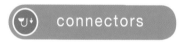

They will show you how to **detox** not just your body, but also your mind and spirit. This is the **wellness approach.**

The term 'wellness' is broad. For some it may mean fitness or food, and others feel it's about better quality sleep, relationships or even work/life balance. It's different for every single person because we are unique. So too are our lifestyles as they are constantly changing. What works for you right now, may not in six months or even next year. We have to be dynamic and so does our 'wellness' approach.

The key to being really well is to stay connected to what's going on in your life; in all areas.

Get to know yourself, love yourself and be able to flex when circumstances call for it. Be mindful of connection - to yourself, your food and the world around you.

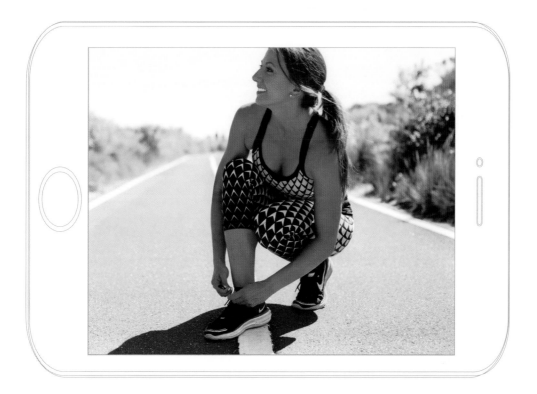

Wellness Loading: Disconnect to Reconnect shows how to just BE, tune in, turn off tech and connect with real food and nature again, through mind and body for an overall detox in the digital era.

Reconnect with your body and live a life of more confidence, inner strength, authenticity and of course; wellness.

Disconnect to Reconnect.

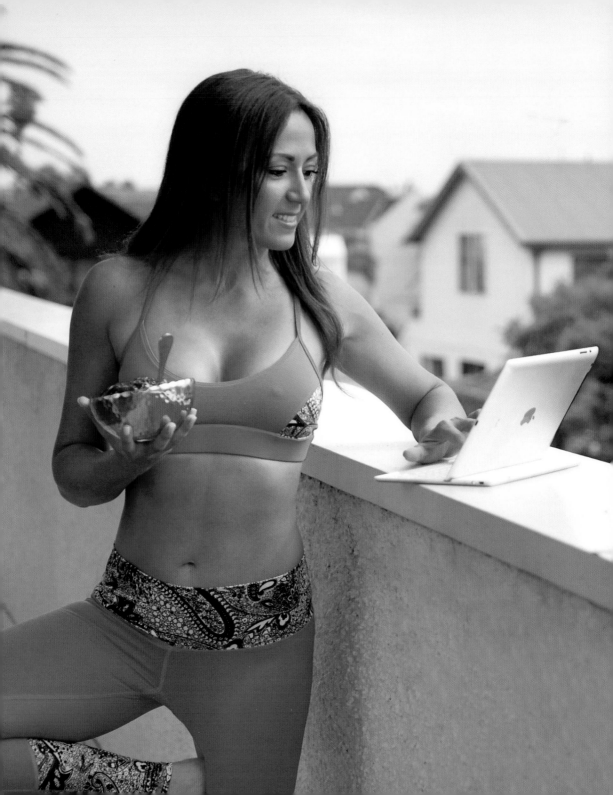

as cliché as it sounds,
it really is all about
#BALANCE

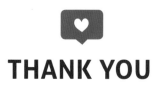

THANK YOU

There are so many people I want to thank for this book. In fact a major part of this title is all about gratitude. I could not be more grateful for all the people that have helped shaped me recently and in turn, inspired me in some way, shape or form to write.

I have observed you and your kindness, lessons, wisdom and love. If I have not mentioned you, then know that if you have been in my life at all, then you have either directly or indirectly been a part of this journey.

To wellness coach, passionate philanthropist, social entrepreneur, and wonderful father, Mike Sherbakov; you taught me more than you realise. When the student is ready, the teacher appears. I will always be grateful to for you inviting me to meet you, your son and your San Diegan tribe in 2015. It made me a better version of myself. I was challenged with many spiritual lessons and exposed to a mecca of wellness within the vortex of energy in San Diego. I'm able to inspire more people now.

To my mum, Terri Lew and her mother, Margot Cohen. Margot may no longer be with us, but she's still with me every time I cook. She taught Mum and I how to create from scratch, using only the most natural ingredients, not letting any part go to waste. Margot's own mother passed away when she was just 12, leaving her to look after her three brothers and sisters, one of whom was a very young infant at the time. She then married at 16 and moved from Morocco to the new state of Israel and took a job cleaning utensils in a hospital. Shortly after, she started her own family, creating four beautiful children with my grandfather Pinchas. My grandparents were hard workers. When they migrated to Australia, I used to pretend I was sick so that Mum would let me stay home with them. As soon I heard Mum's car leave the driveway, I would creep to the kitchen where my grandmother, Margot was cooking and baking - since 5am that morning, mind you! She would turn and say, "Sit down! I know you're not sick. Now be quiet and watch and learn. No writing!" When I cook, I always think of both Terri and Margot.

To my dad, Zelman Lew; thank you for teaching me how to follow my life's dreams. As an artist, you always said to follow my heart, for it knows the way. You've supported me to do this emotionally and physically as a wonderful grandfather, enabling me to work once I became a single mother.

To my ex-husband Warren Sipser, thank you for being my chiropractor and a connected father to our son Beaudy. I love that we teach him how to better love through staying connected as a family.

To Fernanda Ramos, thank you for the wonderful photography you contributed. Your friendship and ability to make me feel relaxed in front of the camera is a gift. I appreciate you.

Dorota Trupp, you are a talented photographer and I'm blessed you have you as a friend. Your food photography shots are spirited.

To Daniel Jorgensen, Colin Gold and Andrew Avi, I was graced with your generosity and talent as photographers.

Rose Parsons, thank you for your hair and make-up on shoots.

Giorgia Maselli, it was a pleasure working with you on some of the food shoots too.

Andi Lew

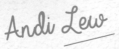

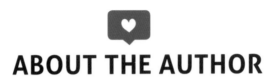

ABOUT THE AUTHOR

A natural nurturer and advocate for healthy living, Andi Lew is a certified Food, Lifestyle and Wellness Coach, renowned Australian TV Presenter and author of five health titles including the three international best sellers, *Eat Fat Be Thin*, *Eat Fat Be Lean* and *Real Fit Food*.

Andi recently spent time in the U.S on a press tour for her fifth book, *Real Fit Food* and appeared on many talk shows across America inspiring people about the real food revolution. This tour moved her to write *'Wellness Loading: Disconnect to Reconnect'* as she observed the prevalence of disconnection among people even as they connected via social media and the World Wide Web.

Andi Lew is a conscious driven mother who cares about community and creating connections. She is a proud mum to her six year old son, Beaudy who inspired her to write her second book, *The Modern Day Mother*, highlighting how "it takes a village to raise a child".

She is a woman on a wellness crusade and has run a cooking school in St Kilda, Melbourne educating thousands of people about food alternatives for people with intolerances. Andi also ran her own wellness centre for over 13 years and is a passionate advocate for holistic health.

Andi is the Food and Fitness coach for Miss Universe Australia and Miss World contestants, creator of vegan protein bars 'Amazebars' and is highly sought after on the daytime TV shows circuit in both America and Australia for her expert advice on wellness and nutrition. She has presented on shows such as *60 Minutes* and *The Today Show*. Andi has also written for magazines such as *Clean Eating Magazine*, *Ultra Fit*, *Australian Natural Health*, *Oxygen* and *Cosmo Pregnancy* and blogged for model mum Miranda Kerr's KORA Organics website.

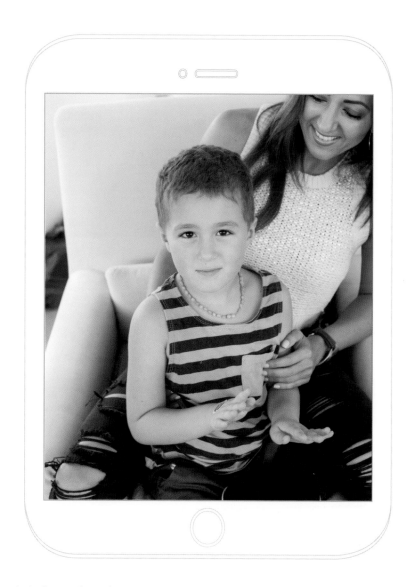

Andi truly believes that when we are happy, at peace and in love with ourselves, then it is easy to want the same happiness, love and peace for others. She hopes her books will provide inspiration to her readers to take charge of their lives by following her holistic approach.

Visit **www.andilew.com** for more information about Andi.

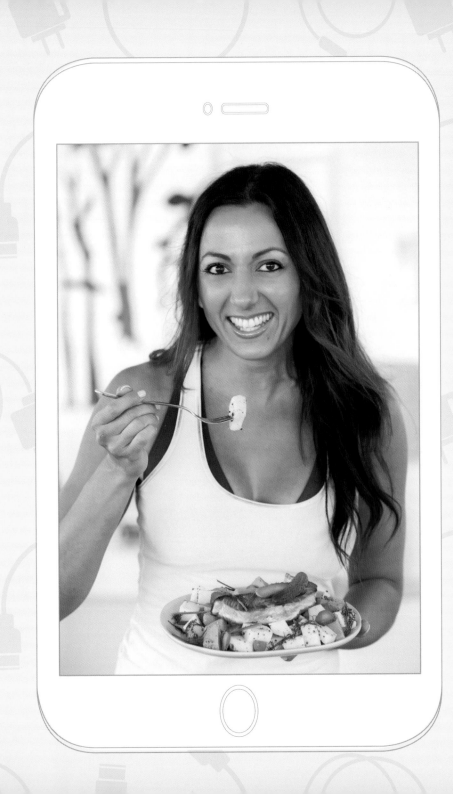

CONTENTS

THE 5 CONNECTORS: HOW TO TURN OFF TECH

CHAPTER ONE

"A human being is a part of the whole called by us universe, a part limited in time and space. He experiences himself, his thoughts and feeling as something separated from the rest, a kind of optical delusion of his consciousness. This delusion is a kind of prison for us, restricting us to our personal desires and to affection for a few persons nearest to us. Our task must be to free ourselves from this prison by widening our circle of compassion to embrace all living creatures and the whole of nature in its beauty." ~ Albert Einstein

How wonderful it is to be able to connect to all living creatures and the wholeness of nature itself! Take for instance the joy the birth of a baby brings, the love of a pet animal, the wonder of magical lightning storms or sunsets and even the smell of rain as it leaves Mother Nature's clouds.

The divine universe we live in has so many gifts for us to share and experience. We know this because the wonderment of a brilliant rainbow that appears in the sky for all to witness, can stop every human in his or her tracks, to observe its gift in the present moment. It's almost like a form of visual meditation that has been designed to enlighten and heighten senses.

Human discoveries have also given us many gifts. Take for instance the invention of aircraft which helped us visit distant family relations, connect with other cultures and experience new sights. The clever creation of the phone, then fax and now computer technology helped us learn and see more.

We have widened our circle and life experiences immensely through the creation of – and connection to – the internet.

Today, we are witnessing a cultural revolution as we increase our connection through technology and social media. Like it or not, this is the way it is. Personally, I have been able to meet new people and find like-minded groups and organisations as a result of our new found social media revolution. I have connected with the most amazing mentors and teachers, journalists, publicists, parents, entrepreneurs and general community as a result of technology. But are we really connected?

Are we turning into an anti-social society? Or can we use this social media revolution to our advantage? Can we take what we need from it, give back to practice gratitude and yet still have balance? How is it possible to look within for the balance, if we are searching for ways to do so on the World Wide Web? You may even be reading this very 'digital detox' book on a device as an e-book. Isn't that ironic? Yet this is ok. We are headed this way, so rather than swim away from the 'computer-era' current, let's work with it to create a way to make it work for us.

As a certified Food, Lifestyle and Wellness Coach, I firmly believe the ticket to personal freedom and wellness lies in my understanding of a holistic approach to life.

Being 'well' is a multi-factorial approach. There's a multitude of things we need to do to create a more vital lifestyle. The key is to start. Because humans love progress. It doesn't matter what our end goal is. If we are progressing, we are going to be happy. Once that ball gets rolling, guess what? You're going to feel more fulfilled, happier and will start to feel more connected!

The term wellness is going to have different interpretations for each person. What makes you well is going to be different to someone else's needs. Our lives are unique and so too are our diets and outlooks, depending on lifestyle and even our genealogy.

There are however, five important discoveries I made that I believe will make a huge difference to your wellbeing and health! But first a little background:

I started lecturing and inspiring others in their workplaces. Big companies such as 'Red Energy' hired me to help their staff achieve balance in their physical lives whilst at the workplace.

Organisations such as Red Energy realised the ramifications of spending eight – or more! – hours a day being sedentary in front of technology. They started taking proactive steps to get their employees moving, be it building a yoga room on site, hiring a massage therapist to visit weekly, investing in staff gym memberships or hiring me to speak to them about their health.

In these seminars, I gave examples of ways of being healthier in a desk job environment. I often recalled my visit to Hylete, a CrossFit apparel company in San Diego, California where I saw staff working at bar stool height desks. This enabled them to stand up and work from their computers which is much better for the cardiovascular system. They also engaged in CrossFit fitness activities during their lunch break. Their productivity was fantastic and the company, even though it was new, grew fast.

In my job as a radio announcer, I saw many Australian radio stations begin to implement the 'bar stool' desk structure too. Using them in the broadcasting area allowed the announcer to stand whilst on air. The added bonus was the fact that when we stand, and not slouch, our voice and energy levels change.

These observations about posture and spinal health as a result of our modern lifestyles concerned me greatly. Using my qualifications as a chiropractor's assistant, I was compelled to create a system of wellbeing that could be applied to our modern 'tech' loaded lifestyle. I'm happy to share it with you right now.

This is where I talk about CONNECTORS and how to 'turn off tech' because it is so important our wellbeing. I also want to make this easy for you.

I want you to start with just one thing. By doing just one thing from my *Wellness Loading* 'Mind and Body Detox Program' for just an hour a day (or for a period of time that you choose) you can then

create a **reconnection** to yourself,
your body and your community.

This is important for we are connected to everything. Let me prove it.

Did you know women report that when they start to spend a lot of time together or reside together, their menstrual cycles start to synchronise? Women also report their menstrual cycle synchronises with the lunar cycle.

Lauren Geertsen, a Nutritional Therapies Practitioner, talks about this very topic in her article published on her 'empowered sustenance' blog. She states:

"Random and uncomfortable periods are the effect of a diet and lifestyle that disconnects us from the rhythm of nature. Modern living means that most women abuse their bodies with various chemicals, antibiotics, prescription medications, the OCP (oral contraceptive pill), extreme emotional stress, the stress of over-exercising, refined foods and more.

Another key factor in hormonal imbalance is artificial light. It widely known that the blue light from electronic device screens disrupts melatonin, wreaking havoc on our sleep cycles. Less well known is that our bodies are so sensitive to light patterns that women can manipulate other hormones by controlling the light at night. This is because our melatonin levels help control the hormones that regulate our periods, according to fertility specialist and author Kate Singer." [1]

We have now learned we are that connected to the earth, the moon and the sun, so that when we try to even change that, our hormones become out of balance. Now that's connection!

What about when birds fly in formation, or a school of fish swim in unison? If one wants to make a turn, does it turn to the others behind and yell, "Hey mate! In 200 metres we'll all turn left, ok?" No they don't. They just do. They know. There's an innate, as well as universal, intelligence guiding us to be the same. Because we are connected.

What about other living creatures? Have you ever noticed how your pet dog follows you around and only decides to fall asleep when you do? And if you permit, usually at the foot of your bed.

What about babies? Did you know that our hearts, breathing and body temperature all synchronise when we co-sleep with our offspring? You only have to look at the works of professor and PHD sleep scientist, James Mckenna, [2] or read *The Science of Parenting* by Margot Sunderland, [3] to find out more about the mutual regulations of parent and child.

The bottom line is; all living creatures are connected. We are designed to be connected to other life. This helps our wellbeing. If you're suffering from depression, doctors suggest you get a cat or dog for companionship – to create a connection.

Living in the big city, and in big houses, far away from each other, we pretend we're alright and don't need anyone's help. Yet we are all suffering on some level, craving connectedness. We used to live in communities, close to each other, caring for one another by taking it in turns to cook, clean and look after children. We hunted together, gathered together and built villages together.

So now we try to create connectedness. Many people have found success in this by practising yoga, meditation, mindfulness and prayer. Yet, when we worked together with nature and in a community that was our yoga and meditation. We connected with each other AND the earth at the same time.

Let's keep going. Here is a perfect example of just how connected we are, even to the planet itself:

Did you know, the percentage of water within our bodies is approximately 70-80%? [4] This is the same percentage in the earth itself. Yes, the earth is about 70-80% water! What is really astounding is that so too are plants! Nourishing our bodies with more plants hydrates us and gives us more life. This is true connection to the earth and environment. Some call this 'mindfulness' or 'mindful eating'. This is one way in which the *Wellness Loading* 'Mind and Body Detox Program' CREATES CONNECTED COMMUNITIES and A HEIGHTENED CONSCIOUSNESS.

Want more stories about connection? I have just a few more:

My son asked me one, "Mum, why does it have to be so windy?" I explained that one of the reasons was to stir and shake things up. Movement is life. For example, the wind moves the water and creates negative ion effects. It moves the trees to shake off dead leaves or drop seeds so more plant life can grow. When water is still, it starts to become murky and dull, even contaminated – in one word, lifeless!

Humans need movement to survive too. As a qualified chiropractic assistant - and having run a wellness chiropractic centre for 13 years - I saw all too well the damaging effects of sedentary lifestyles. Movement also runs the brain. In my chiropractic studies, I learnt the nervous system (our brain) spinal cord and corresponding nerves need clear communication. Misalignment, or 'vertebral subluxation', creates an interference to the nerve system. We need proper movement and nutrition to minimise this.

I draw my final movement point from the phrase "If you don't move, you lose it". That's why when we land in a hospital after an accident, we need a physical therapist to help us move our limbs to stop them from atrophying.

Good chiropractic care can lead to a heightened consciousness and connectedness. It allows us to have clearer communication from brain to body. It helps us to reconnect by removing nerve system interference. With this heightened awareness, we can make healthier choices with a clear head. To find a qualified and registered Chiropractor near you, call the Chiropractor's

Association of Australia, phone: 03 9328 4699.

Now I've shown you how connected we are to our universe, we have finally arrived at the all-important...

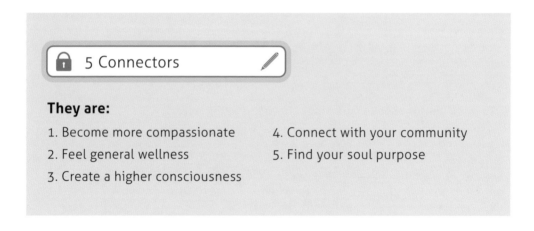

🔒 **5 Connectors** ✏️

They are:

1. Become more compassionate
2. Feel general wellness
3. Create a higher consciousness
4. Connect with your community
5. Find your soul purpose

To achieve the above, you need to do the dreaded: TURN OFF TECH.

Well, I shouldn't really call it 'dreaded'. Let's start by changing our Neuro-Linguistic Programming (NLP). The words we use have a powerful impact on how we feel. Let's focus on what we gain, as opposed to what we feel we will lose. With any addiction, we fear the unknown of what may happen when it's removed from our lives. The phone is a great example. We all know the feeling of **FOMO (Fear of Missing Out)** when we turn it off. We are addicted to the immediacy of the contact. But what if we weren't missing out, but instead gaining, by turning off tech?

Let's make a list of the possible gains:

⊙   better sleep quality

⊙   more clarity

⊕ improved relationships

⊕ improved general feeling 'wellness'

What if we thought a little more left field?

⊕ the possibility of meeting someone in the flesh by looking around you

⊕ improving communication

⊕ less car accidents

⊕ saving battery power

There's so much to gain. I am sure you made a few lists in your head too after being inspired by reading some of the possible gains above.

Did you know that the average person spends approximately four years of his life looking down on his cell phone? Reports have shown that in 2014 there were 1.75 billion cell phone users, and these statistics are on the rise rapidly. [5]

If this doesn't inspire you to turn away from it just a little each day - and start living - then I am not sure what will. A broken device perhaps? Another jest ... but it's funny because it's true though, isn't it?

The good news is, I am not going to make you go cold turkey on me, or even give it up forever! But first, to some background. After returning from a trip to America in October 2015 - where I toured my fifth book *Real Fit Food* - I realised that we, as a society, have become more disconnected when using tech that was supposed to connect us.

In New York, I observed every single person, either scrolling, searching, talking, texting or taking pictures on their devices. At first I wondered if this behaviour was just in the city. People are very productive there. They have high powered jobs, they're ambitious because after all, isn't it the city where dreams are made? People choose to live in New York to dream big, do more and be more, right? So, surely they need their digital devices.

My observation the next day was not in the streets or subways. It was in the local Star Bucks cafe. There was a queue for the bathroom that was 20 people long. Every single person was looking down.

These observations made me miss connection. The last time I had travelled overseas was 13 years prior. I remembered meeting so many amazing people because I was forced to make eye contact and chat to a stranger. I didn't have access to Google maps so I had to stop someone in the street and ask for directions. As for the nearest hotel or restaurant and gym, I could get all that on an app now. Sure it's more convenient now to have that at my fingertips but I missed the connection?

Australia may be less populated but the observations hold true here too. Don't get me wrong. I don't find this new digital age sad. I think it's genius! In fact, if it weren't for apps and social media, I would not have been able to make the many connections I have made over the recent years. I wouldn't have been able to find last minute hotels and accommodations at really affordable rates. Through social media networking, I have met some incredible people, companies and watched some of genius ideas on video blogs. But all this tech has a big downside. It has an immense impact on a vital component to our wellness: our sleep.

Let's talk about the **SLUMP OF SLEEP.** Have you noticed your sleep quality is not what it used to be? Have you ever stopped to count the hours you spend emailing, texting, searching online shopping catalogues or dating apps? How often do you find yourself doing this slumped on the couch at night?

One of my clients, Dr Benjamin Wei, a surgeon, shared some very interesting insights during one of our conversations one day about how technology disturbs our sleep:

"From the beginning of human existence to the discovery of electricity and the creation of light bulbs, humans only exposed to only natural light and no electronic devices, had their circadian clocks synchronised with the rise and fall of the sun. This is how we were created. However, with the advancement of technology and the 24/7 society, we are now altering this nature cycle and this could lead to detrimental consequence to our physical and mental health.

From the very early human existence, the light from the sun tells our body that it is day time. This is achieved by the suppression of the body clock hormone secreted in the pineal gland in our head. The humans then go out to hunt and gather. They then return home when sun is setting and the reduction of the sun light allows the pineal gland to secrete melatonin which makes us feel sleepy. It is the nature's way to tell us, it is time to go to bed and get rest.

Unfortunately, the pervasive glow of electronic devices at night time is disrupting our circadian cycle. The lights from the electronic devices such as computer screens, smartphones and tablets often stay on throughout the night. These devices emit light of all colours but it is the blue spectrum light that suppresses our melatonin production and tricks our brain and body that it is day time. As a result, we are systematically sleep-deprived because of how society works against our natural clocks. Studies have shown sleep deprivation increases the risk of mood disorders such as depression and anxiety and reduces our ability to cope with stress.

Our modern society also encourages children starring at the electronic device screen all night. The danger with disturbing children's sleep is it can affect their brain development. Sleep is important for learning, memory, brain development, health. We're systematically sleep-depriving kids when their brains are still developing, and we couldn't design a worse system for learning.

Many epidemiology studies also demonstrated that shift workers have higher incidence of cancers e.g. breast, colon and prostate cancers). It has been suggested that the disruption of our body biological clock weaken the immune system. Previous animal studies showed that disruption of the biological clock can lead to accelerated neurodegeneration, loss of motor function and premature death.

This is an important issue that people don't talk about because our society is so addicted to 24/7 lifestyle, profit driven society that bombarded us with more electronic gadgets which will result in unintended consequence in the human evolution."

As a wellness coach, I'm all about balance so I'm not advocating a total shutdown from 'screen time'. But I do believe we need to carefully choose the time of day in which we use our technology for the sake of sleep. I suggest considering choosing a number of nights where you do not look at your computer screens or phones right before you go to sleep. I know this might be causing you some panic right now. But believe me, by switching off for just a few nights a week, it will make a difference for you.

It is all about **BALANCE** at nights. If you are going to use **TURN OFF TECH** as one of the 'things' you commit to **TURN OFF TECH** as a part of your *Wellness Loading*, then may I suggest you choose to turn it off at least an hour before retiring? Alternatively, you may choose to not look at devices at all three nights a week for example. The rest of the week, you can look at it all you want, especially if you have a night job that requires you to do so. Just make a plan to turn it off at night a little before bed. Go for it the rest of the time! At least your body will have those quality nights of rest and will adapt.

On the nights you do use tech, I recommend you do something relaxing just before you go to sleep. This allows your brain to start to produce the hormones they need to help you have better quality sleep. When your hormones are happier, your body will work better and in turn, you will be healthier and happier.

Soon I will help you make some goals about how you will go about doing this. You will be able to write down your *Wellness Loading* activities in the back of this book in the journal section.

Now, let's get deeper into the 'WHY' we want *Wellness Loading*. We have explored the benefits for our immediate circle; you. Let's now look at the benefits for our wider circle; our friends, families, loved ones, community and the planet in general. You will be able to start creating a connectedness to the world we live in.

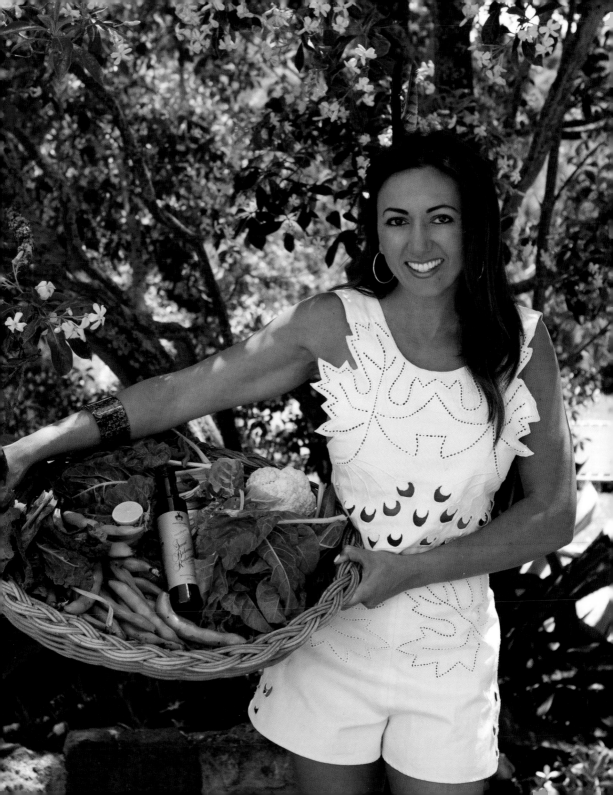

COMPASSION: CONNECTEDNESS TO US AND OUR EARTH

CHAPTER TWO

"The best way to find yourself is to lose yourself in the service of others."
~ Mahatma Gandhi

Have you ever felt lost and disconnected to your soul purpose? Do you ever have moments of wondering you are really here for? Is there something greater you could be doing with your life? Do even know what your soul purpose is? These are profound questions and ones I hope this chapter will help you answer.

We live in a world that has forgotten to serve. Studies show the health benefits of service and volunteer work as it severely decreases stress levels. [1]

To find yourself and feel connected again, means doing two things:

Find your soul's **purpose**
Give back or perform acts of service

As a Wellness Coach, I often get to a great question of my clients, "If you had to wave a magic wand and have a more 'well' life for you, what would that look like?" So let's answer this question together now. Remember: this is with a magic wand so there are no limitations. Freely say and write what you really want!

⊕ **What does your life look like?**

⊕ **What does it feel like?**

⊕ **Describe the days and people in it**

⊕ **Visualise the whole picture**

⊕ **Write all your thoughts down**

Remember, there are no rules. It's your life. They are your dreams and aspirations.

Wellness Coaching is about making small steps to help you achieve your dreams. I am passionate about this role and helping others live their inspired life because I truly believe we are all meant to be doing what we love and loving what we do. For it is when we are 'well' that we are living life with purpose and when we live this way, we are happier. We are at peace and become successful in what we do. We reflect this to others and encourage them to want to do the same.

But the first step is to understand our 'why?' Why do we want to lead this 'well life' that I described above? Your 'WHY' is what will fuel your desire to achieve it.

It's easy to say you want to change but then another year goes by and before you know it, you are still doing the same thing you have always done. You're in a 'hold pattern'.

So now, write down "WHY" a 'well' life is important to you.

Use this statement:

I, *(insert your name)*

....

....

would like to ... *(describe your well life)*

....

....

The most important part of the exercise is next:

So that I can...

....

....

....

....

Many people realise their "So that I can..." reasons look like this:

- ⊛ so that I can spend more time with my children

- ⊛ so that I can open a centre for helping others do the same

- ⊛ so that I can create an animal shelter

- ⊛ so that I can become a teacher that inspires others

You get my drift? These are just some examples to whet your appetite.

Once you have finished writing this, it will then become your mission statement or your **PURPOSE.** When you realise what it is you need to do for your greater soul purpose is when you will have the courage to action it. Type it up or write it up nicely and place somewhere so that you are reminded constantly of your intentions for yourself and for the greater purpose of others.

Humans are designed to serve and love. We feel happier when we do this. Most of the time, we aren't giving enough because we feel we aren't receiving enough. Have you ever heard of the saying "keeping your love tank full"? Let's say you have a tank of love you can fuel others with, but when you've given so much, you may feel empty. This is when we need to start giving back to ourselves.

Write a list of things you can do, to feel more 'full'.

Here are some examples:

- ⊛ light candles
- ⊛ practise yoga
- ⊛ get a massage
- ⊛ listen to relaxing music

- ⊛ watch the sunset or sunrise
- ⊛ paint/colour/draw/do craft
- ⊛ cook
- ⊛ read

- ⊕ garden
- ⊕ play with animals or children
- ⊕ have a pedicure
- ⊕ throw rocks in the ocean
- ⊕ play board games
- ⊕ star gaze

- ⊕ go camping
- ⊕ ride a bicycle to work
- ⊕ meditate
- ⊕ create a vision board
- ⊕ play an instrument

Filling your 'love tank' or wellness cup can also be about gratitude. Some practice 'the art of gratitude'. Gratitude can be a daily thing where you intentionally recognise what you are grateful for. I know some people who jump out of bed each morning and say the things they are grateful for. Some do it at meal time. We have been known to call it 'blessing' the food, as we recognise where it came from and how lucky we are to have it nourish us in such abundance.

Wherever you are in your life, you will always be able to find something to be grateful for because there will always be someone else worse off. Your challenging state cannot remain forever, and while you're in this state, the greatest growth and lessons tend to come forth. It's usually only when we hit rock bottom that the greatest growth comes. We can always be grateful for that and the lessons it brings.

When we are happy within ourselves, we can then be happy for others and want that happiness for others. Because whatever is going on in your world, is not happening to you. You are a reflection of it. How you respond, how you acknowledge, how you perceive and how you receive, is all a reflection of who you are. I have known people in the lowest of lows, or who have so much less than me and yet they are happy, or what I prefer to call; at peace.

How do we achieve happiness within ourselves? How can we be 'at peace'? By living your soul purpose. The very same one you just wrote out. Let's make some small steps toward your above 'Mission Statement'/PURPOSE. What can you do this week to start that ball rolling to help you achieve your soul purpose? Write that down. Start to action it in baby steps. These steps towards your inspired life will help you feel a sense of peace within yourself.

Wellness Coaching is designed to build your self-efficacy and in turn self-confidence, because once you start to see a few small changes working, you will continue. You don't need end results right away but need to see you are progressing. If you are, then you are evolving and creating more happiness and peace.

Have you ever seen the movie, *Pay It Forward* with Kevin Spacey, Helen Hunt and Hayley Joel Osment? It based on the premise of making the world a better place through service and giving. Three kind things are paid forward to three other people and then those three people do the same and so it grows. If you haven't seen the movie, then I suggest you do. It's an oldie but a goodie!

I know of a couple who saw the movie when it first came out in the movie theatre. They decided to pay for the all the people in the next session as an act of paying it forward. A simple act of kindness can make a tremendous impact on a person's life, even your own!

I recently put this theory to the test! This is story about why I was re-inspired to 'pay it forward' with:

One day I invited a friend over to my home for dinner. He had taken me out for numerous meals and I wanted to reciprocate since I am a good cook. Did I just give myself a compliment? Haha! I didn't say I was amazing, but I guess I know what to do after having written three recipe books. I also thought he may really enjoy that act of service and love. However, that night I told him I wanted to find someone that would join me on a wellness crusade. I didn't want a relationship unless someone was going to walk that path with me. He went home and subsequently, we stopped hanging out.

The next morning a magical thing happened. I woke to an email from an incredibly inspiring fellow wellness coach who I had been following on Instagram for about six months. We popped up in each other's feeds in early 2015. He too was admiring my work on Instagram. The email was an invitation to meet with him as he decided he wanted us to connect and collaborate, so he asked if I had plans to visit the U.S. Keep in mind, I had never met this person across the other side of the globe. However, I had researched his work, websites and peers. He was legitimate, however the uncanny timing of the invitation made me feel suspicious. He had also never met me. Why would he want this?

I could not believe what I had read. I blearily re-read the message and then responded, telling him what I had said the night before. My intentions were set, and here he was showing up hours later, presenting me with this opportunity. So many people in Australia had expressed that I should expand my brand to the U.S and this could be my calling. He replied about how it was divine synchronicity and we must trust it. Several messages back and forth were about asking him what his hopes and dreams were for the year and he said to 'love more x100'! I was impressed by someone who wanted to love and serve so deeply. I told him he was amazing and he responded with that I was just a reflection of him.

This statement hit me hard. Aren't we all mirrors of each other? It felt so true to me. The more he radiated love and compassion and kindness, the more I wanted to be those things.

Months passed and we built a stronger connection. I decided to take the leap of faith and take up his offer to stay with him in San Diego so I could meet him and the like-minded folk there. We eventually did connect, collaborate, make magic and inspire each other, but right before I left Australia to meet him, I told him that ever since I had been in regular contact, I was loving and serving more too. He had caused me to want to 'pay it forward' because he was gifting me with a trip to visit. I didn't realise I was going to 'pay' anything forward, but my love tank was full with receiving love and I had gratitude. This opened me up to the following experience:

I was walking down the street with my son after having eaten a late dinner. I saw a homeless man searching through a trash can. Immediately, my intuition told me to go and ask him to a meal. My judgement is usually spot on, but I stood back slightly when asking him so that I could give him the space to consider, and me the space to further make a judgement about safety. He accepted my offer to get a meal together.

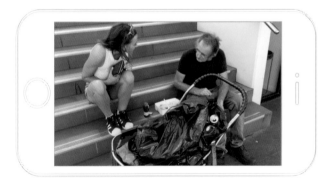

My new friend Trevor ☺

I estimated this man to be in his late sixties. He could have been my father, or anybody's father for that matter. In fact he was somebody's dad wasn't he? As we all walked along the street to a place nearby, he hobbled slowly pushing his life in a trolley. It forced us to slow down, connect heart to heart and we had conversations about the weather that day because it was starting to warm up. I discussed how nice it was to see the sun and he asked how old my boy was and when would he start school. I remember thinking how lovely it was that he asked about my son.

We found a place to eat. He parked his trolley neatly outside and we entered the warm building. People were staring at us but this man is a part of my community and I didn't mind an uncomfortable glare. Then, and after he chose a half a chicken, some rice salad and a chocolate brownie, I told him I should probably get my son to bed. This is where magic happened. He then - wait for it - wished us both well. Hang on a minute! Wasn't I better off than him and meant to be wishing him well? He said he hoped I would find the keys that I lost! I had forgotten that I told him I lost my keys probably at the first restaurant I went to with my son to fill our bellies. I was so surprised. He listened and cared. I discovered that connecting with this new human and being totally present with him for that short period of time had served us both in so many ways, even if just for that moment. My moral of the story? It was mutual.

I told the San Diegan wellness coach this story and felt like my compassion radar was rising tenfold. He said he felt the same. Mirrors? How many more reflections can we create? This is why I am writing now. I trust in you. I trust we can create a more compassionate world and healthier place to live, one act of service at a time, and one act of compassion at a time. This does not have to mean you need to be of service all day, every day. It also does not mean that I believe you should go ahead and invite a homeless man to dinner too! However, this story illustrates how to expand your consciousness to a greater awareness and feeling of love and compassion. When it feels right for you to act upon, you should. But it has to feel right for you. The choice of when, what and how is all yours. The freedom is there. Just expand your awareness to it so that you can create your own acts of service and compassion.

I've talked about being compassion towards others but now I want to turn to the topic of showing compassion for yourself and the earth too. A key way to do this is to begin eating more real, live plants foods. The connection may not be immediately apparent to you but stick with me.

Let's begin with a study published in *Proceedings of the National Academy of Science*. It found that people who walked for 90 minutes in a natural area, as opposed to participants who walked in a high-traffic urban setting, showed decreased activity in a region of the brain associated with depression. It states:

"These results suggest that accessible natural areas may be vital for mental health in our rapidly urbanizing world ... Our findings can help inform the growing movement worldwide to make cities more liveable, and to make nature more accessible to all who live in them." Gretchen Daily, Professor in Environmental Science, Stanford Woods Institute for the Environment. [2]

More than half of the world's population lives in urban settings, and that is forecast to rise to 70% within a few decades. Just as urbanization and disconnection from nature have grown dramatically, so have mental disorders such as depression. City dwellers have a 20% higher risk of anxiety disorders and a 40% higher risk of mood disorders as compared to people in rural areas. People born and raised in cities are twice as likely to develop schizophrenia. [3]

Is exposure to nature linked to good mental health? The researchers in this study postulated that nature does have a beneficial impact on emotion and mood. Furthermore, could exposure to nature help "buffer" against depression? [4] If going for walks amongst nature and plant life helps fight against mental illness, what could actually consuming them do?

I firmly believe humans need to eat more 'live' foods. If you can kill it or grow it, you should eat it! This doesn't mean your diet has to be animal-based, but is about eating foods that are real and alive as opposed to eating packaged and processed foods. If you'd like to know more about this important topic, my fifth book, *Real Fit Food*, deals with this extensively. The more alive the food is, the more life it gives us and the more nutrition it has. It is the micro-nutrition (vitamins and minerals) that helps us feel full. As the name suggests, processed foods have been through a 'process', with all the micro-nutrition stripped from them. That is why when we consume these products, we never feel like we have had enough and are always looking for that 'something else'.

So let's ingest this life force, because plants not only have nutrition that we need to act as medicine in our bodies, but they also actually contain something really vital for wellness: water! As I mentioned at the start of this book, just like us, plants contain about 70-80%

water? Some plants contain up to 90%. [5]

Generally speaking, our race is becoming chronically dehydrated from the over-consumption of highly processed sugary and salty food. Rehydrating with water is important but we can up that through our food intake too. Plants will do this. Are you starting to see the connection between us and plants?

EAT MORE PLANTS

You don't have to be a complete vegetarian or vegan to benefit (although making that decision is fantastic for your health!). By simply incorporating some more foods that are 'alive' into your diet, you will not only benefit physically but will also help create a better planet, reducing your carbon footprint by eating less meat.

Brock Bowen, a 'Lifetarian' shared this with me during one of our conversations:

"In our modern society eating has become a fast paced, mindless, empty, low value part of life. Fast food, microwave meals, factory farmed meats and processed food like substances. Fruits and vegetables remind us to slow down, to connect with the source of our food and the farmers who prepare it for us. As this mindfulness grows deeply within us, our compassion for all of life returns. This is part of the enchantment of life."

Do you know what's really interesting? Many of us think we only get protein from animal sources. I know I did before I started researching. When want to include protein in our meals, we immediately think of meat. However, vegetables and plants like cacao (the raw unrefined version of chocolate) contain protein too.

Some vegetables highest in protein are:

⊙ Broccoli

⊙ Peas

⊙ Kale

⊙ Mushrooms

⊙ Asparagus [6]

Their protein content isn't as high as an animal source, but the more plants you eat and the wider the variety, the more nutrition you receive, helping with digestion and a multitude of other benefits. For example, eating greens help us to easily digest animal protein as they're alkalizing. This is why some protein powders are made from Pea Protein Isolate. The online raw foods retailer, Amazonia do an amazing plant based protein, with equally high bio-availability. It's also combined with pre-biotics to help with healthy gut function and absorption of nutrients.

Eating more plant foods will maximize your nutritional intake. We need macro-nutrition (fats, carbohydrates and proteins) but also micro-nutrition (vitamins and minerals) to help us feel full. The amygdala is the part of the brain responsible for switching off our hunger mechanism when it is full on a nutritional level. This part of the brain doesn't care about portions. It cares about types of calories - and that is nutritional content from real/whole food sources. If you eat nutrient dense foods, you will feel full.

Processed food lacks nutrition and is packed with salt and sugar. The processing also removes good fats that are imperative for hormonal and nerve system health. These systems are made up of fats so we need to fuel them with just that. Good fats are those from plant source foods like seeds, avocado, nuts and coconut.

If you have brain fog from too much tech, remove it with proper hydration and plant-based foods. I hope I've shown you plants are a key nutrient in feeding our brains. They can act as medicine.

Finally, I'm not going to prescribe a diet because, first of all I am not qualified to be prescriptive. Even if I was, each person is too unique. The key is to be more **CONNECTED** to your body and lifestyle. Be compassionate to yourself through the food you consume and to others, through your actions. This should be your running theme.

THE WELLNESS CONCEPT: RECHARGE WITH SUPERFOODS AND HYDRATION

CHAPTER THREE

"Health is a state of body. Wellness is a state of Being."
~ J. Stanford

We touched on what wellness is in the previous chapters and how it's more than just having health. Let's now delve into fully understanding the term 'wellness'. The difference between 'sick care' and 'well care'.

WELLNESS IS A PARADIGM SHIFT

Wellness is about being proactive, not reactive. Rather than wait until you are unwell, it is easier to stay well. Don't "wait 'til it's broke to fix it."

The allopathic model, or medical model, works on the philosophy that you wait until something is wrong and then you react. It is mechanistic in its approach as it looks straight at the symptom, often failing to acknowledge connection between mind, body and spirit. Let's take tonsillitis for example. The medical model says we need to remove the part that is not well. Conversely, the wellness model understands we are connected to our bodies – and to even the earth itself – so it seeks address the cause of the condition. The wellness model wants to know why that part of the body got sick. Only then will it attempt to address the tonsillitis. The wellness model is a holistic approach, believing the body, when sick, is merely in a state of unbalance. By bringing a balance back to our mind and body, we can create better health again, emotionally and physically, because remember that too, is connected. It's preventative in its approach.

So wellness is about being proactive. In fact, by being proactive when it comes to health, you may even increase your quality of life. Prevention is better than cure. In fact, prevention is the cure.

PREVENTION IS THE CURE

There is a revolution taking place, and you are part of it. We live in a time where people openly question medical authorities because as whole, we seem to be getting sicker. Health care costs are rising beyond the ability of most individuals and even governments to pay. The physical, social and financial costs are just too high, and spiralling further out of control. The current generation wants to take back control of their own health, thus the wellness revolution was born. We are in it.

I've come to this realisation after much research where I found the third leading cause of death in the Western World, is preventative medical or hospital error. By the time we get sick and land up in the hands of a doctor at a hospital, the chances are very high that there will be a mistake. The 'right drugs at the wrong time' or the 'wrong drugs at the right time'.

No matter how advanced medicine becomes, sometimes waiting for symptoms to appear before reacting is just too late. Studies performed in 2013 show that we can't always rely on the medical model to save us. While chemical and surgical intervention movements have been highly successful for many years, they've failed to deliver what we all hoped and believed they could give us - health. [1] This has led to a boom in the wellness industry as millions seek answers for themselves; exploring alternative therapies, attending seminars, buying books on healing and searching for answers on the World Wide Web.

There may come a time where you need to go to a health professional as we develop chronic conditions. We may have neglected certain signs or symptoms and you may need their expertise to help guide you back to health. If you choose the right health care professional, the best thing about them is they can monitor your progress and they can hopefully educate you on what wellness is. I say 'hopefully' because the true meaning of the word 'doctor' means 'teacher'.

"The doctor of the future will give no medication, but will interest his patients in the care of the human frame, diet and in the cause and prevention of disease."
Thomas Edison

Mr Edison's word echo loudly in my ear when I think about the Chiropractic industry. Chiropractors are focused on wellness and holism. They restore the health of the human frame through removing nerve system interference with gentle, safe and scientific adjustments. They acknowledge the nervous system is the master controller of every cell, tissue and organ in our body. When your nervous system (brain and spinal cord and nerves that branch off that) are working with clearer signals, then that helps regeneration to occur and your system works optimally.

But let's bring us back to the now. What can you do today to increase the quality of your life tomorrow? So many illnesses are created today, as a result of our lifestyles; stress related illness, heart disease, diabetes, even cancer. They're because of the life choices we are making. Let's take a stomach ulcer for example. It appears as a result of certain medications, alcohol, smoking and even, stress. Amazing that negative thoughts can create this![2] But the very same thoughts can remove it. Well not exactly the same, because they will obviously be more positive and relaxed thoughts to remove a stomach ulcer!

I have heard of many cancer survivors who have focused their minds on removing certain types of cancer through the power of positive thinking. Brandon Bays is a perfect example. The American author and alternative therapist is known worldwide for her book, *The Journey*, a life-healing guide. It is the story of her battle with a basketball sized tumour which she conquered and removed without invasive surgery or drugs in just six and a half weeks, amazing herself and her doctors.

Brandon Bay's example does not mean that this path is for everyone. However, making positive health changes can only benefit you and at the very least, if it increased the quality of your life by even 1%, surely you would try it? If you found out you had cancer, what would you do to radically change your life? Most cancer survivors report that they have made several changes, to be able to go into remission. Most of them include things like nutrition and alkalized water.

Would you:

⊙ Improve your diet?

⊙ Meditate?

⊙ Listen to music?

⊙ Take up a hobby?

⊙ Spend more time with loved ones?

⊙ See an integrative health care specialist?

⊙ Take up yoga or a sport?

⊙ Drink more water?

⊙ Breathe more and think less?

⊙ Unplug digital devices?

⊙ Rest and rejuvenate?

THEN WHY ARE YOU NOT DOING THAT NOW? Why wait for cancer or illness to occur? This is the wellness approach. Wellness is proactive, rather than reactive. Let's get started and implement this approach into your life. Please note: do not try and do everything at once. This is not the wellness approach. FIND BALANCE. This is not a quick fix diet detox plan. Wellness or *Wellness Loading* is a lifestyle that you want to keep implementing for years to come.

Usually when we go on a diet, we go all in. This is then followed up by doing nothing. Then we need to go back on the 'all' diet again and only to be followed by nothing - which usually means you don't do anything about your health as you know what lies ahead: the diet again! I think you can tell I'm not a fan of the 'all or nothing' approach!

The wellness approach is about being able to sustain healthy choices. It is the choices you make today that determine the quality of your life tomorrow. Time is precious. Caring for your health when you already have it will not only improve the quality of your life, it will prolong it. If you think you haven't the time to exercise, to see a preventative health practitioner or to chop up vegetables instead of microwaving a meal, just realise that the time you are 'saving' will simply be subtracted from your life at its end.

⊙ To realise the value of ONE YEAR, ask a student who has failed a grade or a cancer patient with a year to live.

⊙ To realise the value of ONE MONTH, ask a mother who has given birth to a premature baby.

- ⊕ To realise the value of ONE WEEK, ask the editor of a weekly newspaper.

- ⊕ To realise the value of ONE DAY, ask a daily wage labourer with children to feed.

- ⊕ To realise the value of ONE HOUR, ask the lovers who are waiting to meet.

- ⊕ To realise the value of ONE MINUTE, ask a person who has missed the train.

- ⊕ To realise the value of ONE SECOND, ask a person who has avoided an accident.

- ⊕ To realise the value of ONE MILLISECOND, ask the person who has just won a silver medal in the Olympics.

- ⊕ To realise the value of ONE INSTANT, ask the chiropractor who just released the life trapped by a bone on a nerve. [3]

People ask me all the time how I stay inspired to be well. I then say, does highlighting how much our time is limited help you? The average person lives to the age of about 82. That's 82 summer seasons. How old are you now? How many summers have you got left? How would you like to live those?

"The most unexpected thing that happens to us is old age."
Count Leo Tolstoi

Besides thinking about time, I educate myself about what the body does and how it responds to certain foods. I surround myself with like-minded people to stay inspired and encourage support. Finally, I allow myself to be real, or be human, and make mistakes. I love to just let go and have fun now and then. But then, I get back on the track.

In order to create connection to inspire wellness, we must make a choice to disconnect from our device and reconnect with an inspiring food choice at meal times. Food is not just nourishment for the body, but also our minds and souls. Humans are naturally excited by colour and variety, so choosing a mixture of colourful, fresh foods to eat – and enjoying the creative cooking process itself – can bring about a sense of connection and peace.

Here's a great example of this: I had a very busy surgeon come to me for wellness coaching and he decided he wanted to eat better because of his hectic schedule. We had some private cooking lessons but I also suggested a couple of online organic food companies he could order from. He insisted on doing another six weeks of cooking classes because he felt a reconnection to the food in making and creating of it and it made him feel 'more' well. Isn't that amazing? He had limited time in his day, but cooking helped him feel relaxed. It was only one day a week he decided to cook, but it was his special day to reconnect through this means.

charge your device, walk away
and **recharge** yourself

This sections deals with being proactive with our wellness and **CREATE** supercharged **GENERAL WELLNESS** through eating superfoods and hydrating properly!

Eating superfoods will give you optimal nutrition for longevity and health. This can go a long way in helping to cure our technological addictions. The more satisfied we feel through nutrition, the more satisfied we can start to feel in our general health. Creating feelings of satisfaction in other areas of your life, helps you feel more balanced, centred and less in the need of searching for that 'something else' – which more often than not comes in the form of a hand-held device!

Loading wellness is a mind, body and spirit connection. The yogis have this down pat. They know when you are flexible in your body, you're also flexible in your mind. Your physiology creates a change in emotional status. Addressing the root again, can help our 'whole' be healthy.

Before we get right into superfoods, let's explore a little about why it may be a good idea to do a little detox. Why would we bother with a cleanse? There are so many toxins in our world that they can be hard to avoid. There's a pill for every ill – and a corresponding set of side effects. Other stressors on our bodies include: pollution, passive smoking and carcinogens in personal hygiene products (you can actually get some great products without nasties but that's a whole other chapter! In fact, it's another book: *7 Things Your Doctor Forgot to Tell You* which I co-authored with Dr Warren Sipser).

> "Life is like a tree and its root is consciousness.
> Therefore, once we tend the root, the tree as a whole will be healthy."
>
> Deepak Chopra

Gut health is paramount for wellness. Our guts are our second brain, so we need to not only feed it properly but we may also need to repair it. Repair it with pro-biotics and pre-biotics and follow up with a good bone broth. There's a great recipe for bone broth in *Eat Fat Be Lean*, a book I co-authored with Dr Natalie Kringoudis. Use organic apple cider vinegar in the bone broth, which is really just the old fashioned chicken soup grandma used to make. There's a good reason why they call it the "Jewish Penicillin"! The vinegar draws collagen from the bones and collagen repairs tissue. That helps heal the gut wall, in case you have leaky gut syndrome and don't know it. We are all prone to leaky guts because medications damage our gut health.

Our gut is also exposed to an everyday build-up of caffeine, alcohol and processed foods. This all impacts upon our very sensitive organs and immune systems. Side effects can be feeling tired, stressed, skin breakouts, excess weight and even weakened immune systems.

Our immune systems may be low for more than one reason:

- ⊙ stress

- ⊙ interference to the nerve system

- ⊙ poor gut health, including leaky gut syndrome

- over-medicating and other toxins like smoking, alcohol and other drugs

- poor nutrition, by eating refined foods and not enough organic/whole and nutrient dense foods

- lack of sleep

- environmental toxins

- exposure to electronics. Time in front of screens (like cell phones, televisions, computer screens, video games, close to electronic equipment, or close to electric power cables. These all emit electromagnetic fields which can be detrimental to our health if over-exposed.)

All of these stressors can contribute to a free radical process. Free radicals are molecules, and all molecules have electrons; they repel or attract. In the case of free radicals, they have a free limb/electron.They seek out other electrons from other molecules to stabilise themselves. Sound too technical? Bear with me. In this process, it tends to destabilise that molecule and the free radicals create a chain reaction and other free radicals. Think about the little dudes in a conga line, causing damage wherever they go. They damage lipoproteins and unsaturated fatty acids in cell walls, which can impair cell function. Conventional wisdom states free radicals cause ageing, and in turn an oxidative stress process. Over the past few decades, extensive research has been carried out about how this process less to disease and inflammation. Oxidation is thought to be increased by the above mentioned stressors. But our bodies also have the natural ability to combat free radical defences. Free radicals damage our cellular molecules at a greater rate than our body can produce. Antioxidants, which squelch the reactivity of these highly reactive molecules, are one way to slow the ageing process and increase general wellness. Vitamin E in particular has been found to reduce oxidative stress associated with diabetes.

Thankfully, we have our own naturally occurring antioxidant systems and detoxification systems that can neutralise free radicals or clear toxins from the body. These are things like Glutathione. Technical, I know, but we will also get into the dietary forms of antioxidants soon. These are the ones we can add to our wellness cup!

Cleansing and detoxing is a perfect way to boost detoxification systems, flush out toxins, hydrate cells, boost immunity and of course, nourish your body with super nutrition. Start by removing nerve system stimulants like caffeine, or alcohol and drugs, smoking or even passive smoking or other toxins. Start consuming more nutrient dense foods, like superfoods that are plant derived. At the very least, eating more fruits, vegetables, nuts, seeds, herbs and other plant foods which will be a great form of detoxing your body. Most whole foods will have some sort of compound that will act as an antioxidant or work to support one.

Antioxidant rich foods, otherwise known as superfoods, include:

⊛ orange or yellow whole foods like carrots, sweet potatoes, rockmelon and capsicums

⊛ dark coloured fruits like berries, cherries, prunes and dates

⊛ bioflavonoids found in vegetables and dark berries

⊛ buckwheat and soba noodles made from buckwheat

⊛ garlic and onions

⊛ citrus fruits

⊛ broccoli, cauliflower and Brussel sprouts (cruciferous vegetables). These may be useful in cancer prevention

⊛ edamame and legumes

⊛ miso and green tea

⊛ oily fish that are high in essential fatty acids (mackerel, sardines and Atlantic salmon).

⊛ plant based 'good-fat' foods like nuts and seeds, tahini (made from crushed sesame seeds), avocados and flaxseed oils or coconut oil

⊖ herbs and spices, especially turmeric which is a great natural anti-inflammatory

Some foods give you more bang for your buck, but a variety of nutrition is always key. Some foods may contain higher levels of vitamins than others. For example, red capsicum contains three times the amount of Vitamin C (170mg) than an orange (52mg) and guava even more (240mg).

The extra bonus of eating these whole foods rich in antioxidants can be for your mind. The principles behind veganism, or plant eating are 'Eating Consciously and Compassionately'. I term this MINDFUL EATING. You are being mindful with your food choices and can get connected again to yourself and nature. The largest benefit to eating more plants or living a vegan lifestyle is about increasing awareness. It's about realising where your food comes from, what it takes to get it to your plate and how animal food production impacts other creatures and our environment. It's also awareness about how certain foods 'feel' in our bodies and how they influence our mood. Though a plant-based diet isn't a magic cure against normal emotions like anger and depression, many people do testify they feel much better and more positive once embracing a vegan diet. It gives you a different outlook towards the world around you and also makes you appreciate the beauty of nature's finest foods. It's about living in a kinder manner rather than killing other creatures just for the sake of a burger or piece of chicken with cheddar cheese fries on the side. It's about making the connection.

As an aside: you don't have to go totally 'meat-less' to achieve wellness. If you do choose to eat an animal, make sure it has had a proper quality of life; it was free to roam and was not fed with hormones and antibiotics. Just being organic will not be enough, so read packaging very carefully. This is another way of being mindful of your choices.

Now that you have all this information about what foods do what and how your body responds, I think it's easier to stay inspired to make more positive eating choices.

Wellness Loading is all about cooking and preparing foods that don't use the technology of a microwave. Eat raw in summer if your gut can handle it or gently warm foods over a flame on the stove or in a gas, or electric oven. Microwaves can remove the nutrition. How on earth do you eat this way, I hear you ask? I get it. You're busy with a family and your job. I am too. So I have created recipes to get you inspired to start eating more plants along with your other foods. All the recipes are super quick, easy and very tasty. In fact, the kids may even be able to help you in the kitchen! Getting your children to help you is another way of re-connecting. There's something about the art of creating meals with family, friends and loved ones. It's combining the art of being with nature and nurturing yourself and others.

People often ask why my son is able to avoid junk foods, because they find it challenging to get their kids interested in healthy food. I know all mothers have lots of different ways that work for them, but my top five tips are:

⊛　Monkey see, monkey do

Let your child see you enjoy eating whole foods and avoiding processed foods. They are learning from you every minute of each day and they want to be just like you.

⊛　Try to breastfeed full term if possible

The World Health Organisation's current guidelines suggest "two years and beyond." After the age of 12 months, when solids are present in the child's diet, the immune cells and antibodies increase in the breast milk, meaning that human milk is designed to be more than just nutrition. It's nutritional medicine. Human milk, designed for humans, creates immunity, analgesia and so much more. The feedings become less frequent and they're more efficient. Whilst I understand it may not be possible or fit everyone, I have witnessed this can help a child be more interested in whole foods and be less addicted to processed foods. They get a taste of a larger variety of whole foods through your milk. May I suggest you read any book by top Lactation Consultant, Pinky McKay for more information? She's a bestselling author and all of her books are of value. I was honoured to have her write the foreword to my second book, *The Modern Day Mother.*

⊛　Get your child to help you in the kitchen

Getting them involved in the making of the food, will encourage them to eat it. If they feel they have contributed to the process and creation, they're more likely to try something new.

⊛　Have FUN creating the meal!

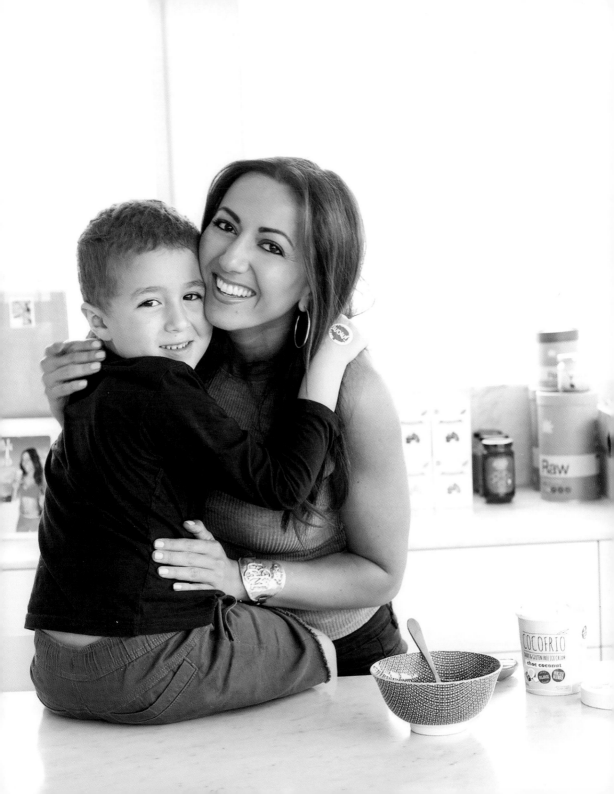

It's great to get the kids helping you create the meal but for it to really work, you HAVE to make it fun! Try to encourage them by giving lots of compliments. Tell them how good they are and how proud you are of them for trying. Tell them how much you appreciate their help and how it makes you feel to see them learning something new.

⊙ Make it tasty!

Perhaps trial the recipe on yourself first so that you know it will taste good and it will work. If it doesn't or you don't have time for that, remember that the experience of 'failing' is only going to bond you more. There isn't winning and losing, only winning and learning. This is a martial arts philosophy I love to practice in my everyday life too. All my recipes are easy to do with kids and use alternatives to sugars, wheats and dairy so that they're still tasty.

SUPERFOODS

The more superfoods you can incorporate into your day, the more wellness you can create. Superfoods are foods that have more nutrition in them than other types of food. They're so nutrient dense, that you feel satiated for much longer. Over-processed foods may make you feel restless as a result of inflammation they can cause in your gut. The artificial additives or colourings (chemicals) can contribute to feelings of ill health and lack of wellbeing.

The more we load our bodies with whole, live, real foods, the more we will crave those. Low calorie, over-processed foods may make us feel initially full, but are we really full? Sometimes it can be a case of 'fake full' - bloated and loaded up with 'empty calories' that aren't serving our bodies with nutrition which translates into wellness. It leaves us only searching for that 'something else' again.

So we are beginning to learn that 'feeling full' and 'feeling satiated' are two different things? Your brain will only switch off its hunger mechanism when it is feeling satiated nutritionally. Your brain knows what types of nutrition you've received that day, week or month, and what you're missing. This is why when you eat real, whole, live foods and foods that are rich in nutrition - like superfoods - you will feel more content.
Some amazing superfoods are now available almost everywhere. There are health food

aisles popping up in major supermarkets, but my favourites are from Power Superfoods, because they're organic and very high quality (see www.powersuperfoods.com).

Cacao powder

Please note this is not the same as Cacoa. The difference is where the 'a' and the 'o' are placed. Cacao is the raw, unprocessed version of the Cacoa. The one that isn't processed; Cacao, is rich in magnesium and protein. It does have a bitter taste, but you can easily sweeten it with sugar alternatives like plant based Stevia, xylitol, coconut sugar, coconut syrup, coconut flower nectar and rice malt syrup, which are all much more lower GI (Glycemic index). If you don't have a weight or hormonal issue, you can sweeten your Cacao in recipes with honey, or coconut syrup and maple syrup or agave nectar.

Chia Seeds

Chia seeds are probably one of the most nutrient dense superfoods that exist. They are the highest known plant source of Omega-3, with eight times more than salmon! The Omega-3 fatty acid is very stable in chia seeds because of its powerful naturally occurring antioxidants.

Other nutrients present in chia seeds are zinc, folate, iron, magnesium, B12 and calcium. Most people don't know what to do with Chia seeds other than sprinkle them on salads and put them in smoothies, so I have a few recipes for you in Chapter 5.

Super Fruits and Berries

Goji, Acai, Lucum fruit, Maca and other ancient berries are rich in antioxidants and Vitamin C. You can get them from incredible companies like Power Superfoods and Amazonia. When we flood the body with antioxidants, we fight the free radicals and combat oxidative stress. Doing this helps slow ageing and creates wellness. Put them in any recipe or eat them with a handful of nuts and seeds.

Seaweeds

Dulse, Wakame Flakes and Nori are all types of superfood seaweeds that many other cultures have been enjoying for hundreds of years. This is one reason why the Japanese look so young! Their diet consists of good fats which are imperative for feeding the hormones and nervous system. The Japanese also consume a lot of seaweed which contain a huge amount of antioxidants. Dulse seaweed for example is a natural treasure chest of goodness, with Vitamins A, B1, B2, B3, B6, B12, C, and E, and minerals like potassium, calcium, magnesium, phosphorous, chromium, iodine and zinc and trace elements. I love to sprinkle them on potato salads and eggs or avocado.

The recipes in the back of this book include some of these antioxidant rich foods and superfoods to help you feel more connected to your body and the earth. If you make them with your family or loved ones, hopefully you will be also creating a digital detox for more than just you! I know all too well how hard it is to get the iPad away from the little guy, especially if he has witnessed working on it, but stopping for meal times to reconnect is wonderful, even if only once a day or every second day!

HOLY HYDRATION - CONNECT WITH YOUR COMMUNITY

Water is absolutely essential to the human body's survival. A person can live for about a month without food, but only a week without water. Water helps to maintain healthy body weight by increasing metabolism and regulating appetite. Water also helps to increase energy levels.

As a rule, we aren't consuming enough water. Adult bodies are made up of approximately 72% water and we lose around 12 cups a day through normal activity. We need to replace that water loss for healthy bodily functions to occur. This replacement should not include caffeinated drinks like tea or coffee as they do not adequately replace water loss. I was surprised when I recently learned that this is not common knowledge. A friend told me she thought she was hydrating properly but was counting her coffee and tea drinks as a cup.

The most common cause of daytime fatigue is actually mild dehydration. A mere 2% drop in body water can trigger:

- ⊙ trouble with basic math

- ⊙ difficulty focusing, fatigue and yawning

- ⊙ erratic and moody behaviour

- ⊙ constipation

- ⊙ aches and pains unrelated to injury/infection

- ⊙ craving for sugar, sweets and caffeine

Dehydration is a condition in which the body's ability to operate as a self-healing organism is blocked. It affects blood pressure, blood-sugar metabolism, digestion and kidney function. Fatigue and headaches are the first symptom of dehydration. Constipation is also common.

You would think that our body would tell us when we are thirsty. But the modern world's obsession with coffee, soft drinks, fruit juice, processed foods and additives has desensitised our thirst mechanism. We have forgotten what it feels like to be thirsty. We often mistake it for hunger and we reach for a coffee, sugary drink - or even a digital device - before reaching for water.

Studies show that 75% of Americans are chronically dehydrated and this statistic is likely applicable to much of the world's population. In 37% of Americans, the thirst mechanism is so weak that it is often mistaken for hunger. Lack of water is the number one trigger for daytime fatigue. [4]

It takes four to six weeks to rehydrate the body properly - it needs to be coaxed out of dehydration mode, which is the water equivalent of starvation mode. The primary goal of the body is survival. When a body has remained dehydrated for long enough, it will retreat into survival instinct, storing water for the future. It takes some time before the body trusts that the period of chronic dehydration has come to an end.

This information shows us the 'holiness' of proper hydration. If you're still not sure, keep this little mantra in mind: Reach for the drink of life, not the device! Hydration will provide you with increased energy and vitality. It can support a whole health strategy for a longer, healthier life. It will help you feel more connected to your body and even your mind.

Water is present in whole foods. Processed foods have no water content. Let's look at sugar as an example. At one point, it was a whole food as sugar comes from sugar cane. Sugar cane is raw, whole and unprocessed. Chewing this cane is fantastic but it takes a little getting used to. It also contains other nutrients such as fibre. You can take the juice out of the sugar cane and it will be sweeter. You can dry the juice out of it and it will be sweeter again (taking the water out dilutes it). This description is the start of 'process' of creating sugar; taking the WATER out of it as a whole food. We then get raw sugar, then white sugar, then castor sugar, then icing sugar as it becomes finer, sweeter and more highly processed. The processing technique uses heat to burn off all the nutrients – nutrients we need to keep us full. It's no longer a real food. It's no longer a whole food. Had we chewed on the sugar cane, we would have been more satiated and felt fuller quicker. This is but one example of how the 'processing' of whole foods sucks all the life-giving water out of them and can even turn them into a chemical cocktail.

I've talked about why water is so important but what is the right water to drink? Water that is alkaline is best and of the highest quality. Drinking alkalized water helps neutralise acids and restore health. Alkaline water also creates the correct structure and energy to allow for cellular hydration. Water must have the right properties to allow the body to hydrate properly, mimicking what Mother Nature does so well.

There are so many benefits to alkalized water but instead of listing them all, I invite to you to visit www.zazen.com.au to find out more about their 'Alkaline Water System'. You can easily get a filter system installed in your home. If this doesn't suit you, you can also buy bottled alkalized water from companies that are community driven and consciously making the world a better place by giving back.

Generosity Water is one such company. They sell alkalised water to developed nations and use their profits to provide drinking water to developing nations. A wonderful use of the 'pay it forward' philosophy! The founder of the company, Jordan Wagner, is an amazing entrepreneur. He was raised in Los Angeles and began his first business at age 14. After visiting East Africa in 2008, Jordan was inspired to use his business acumen to make a global impact. In just five years, he's led the non-profit organisation *www.generosity.org* to raise $4 million to bring clean water to over 300,000 people in 19 countries.

Jordan also produced the critically acclaimed documentary *La Source* narrated by Don Cheadle, and was named 'Humanitarian of the Year' by The Small Business Council of America in 2013. He has been a featured speaker at a number of elite leadership events including Deepak Chopra's Leadership Summit and is committed to seeing his generation make a positive impact on the world today.

Generosity Water are also committed to the environment so all bottles are made from 100% recycled materials, keeping plastic out of landfills and putting it to good use! A large proportion of their profits are put towards water solutions around the world. There are currently 768 million people in the world that do not have access to clean drinking water, and each year this crisis kills more people than war, AIDS and famine combined.

Need more reasons for drinking water? I've given you a lot! It connects you to your body and can also provide you a chance to give back to our world, as Generosity Water's example shows.

There is one last way to stay inspired and be well. It's that magic word 'gratitude'. When we are grateful for what we have (the water we have to drink) when some don't have it all, it changes our perception on nourishment. Be in a space of gratitude when eating well, thinking about your health and wellness and the quality of hydration we have access to. The 'attitude of gratitude' is immensely powerful. Let's move to the next chapter with this in mind.

KNOW YOURSELF, LOVE YOURSELF: CREATE A HIGHER CONSCIOUSNESS

CHAPTER FOUR

*"When asked what gift he wanted for his birthday, the yogi
replied: I wish no gifts, only presence." ~ Unknown*

I love this famous quote by Bil Keane: *"Yesterday's the past, tomorrow's the future, but today is a gift. That's why it's called the present."* Being in the now is where we find peace. I call it the 'heart of love'. Are you ready to receive the true gift of presence so that you can create more wellness in your life?

Think about the experience of your first kiss with someone. Didn't it feel like time was standing still? You have the same feeling when you hold a baby in your arms. No matter whose baby it is, you feel the whole world melt way as they look up at you with their little eyes. You can't help but get lost in their little features, marvelling at their tiny hands, tiny feet and tiny nose. You are totally present in that moment of love. This is why I call being present 'heart of love'.

Yoga, meditation and prayer are three practices we can use to achieve this 'present' state. Yoga is centred on quieting the mind. Concentrating on poses while focusing on the breath clears the mind. It also helps the body shift out of 'fight or flight mode'. During this mode, the body releases an abundance of hormones that are detrimental to our overall wellbeing if they occur continuously. With the way we run our lives today, we seem to be in a permanent state of 'flight or fight'! Excess adrenalin and cortisol is released in this mode, creating an acidic environment in the body. This can be breeding ground for things like cancer. Yoga is one way to combat this.

Yoga poses that are especially challenging also help you to learn more about yourself, your limitations and unconscious beliefs about yourself. You may think "I feel so weak. I can't do this" or "I want to give up." How often in your day-to-day life do you talk to yourself this way? Practices such as yoga will help you become aware of these thoughts and any unconscious thought patterns you are you holding on to. You can discover any self-limiting beliefs you may have unconsciously created.

Practising yoga may not be for everyone but it is the art of 'being still' I want you to focus on. Other thoughts may creep in during this time but this is normal. Like anything, it does take practice to quieten your mind, allow the love in and release the thoughts of past and future. Even if you aren't successful to begin with, you will get there. At least you've tried so you're further ahead than anyone who isn't trying all!

Your effort to become a better version of yourself will be rewarded just by trying. When I was learning martial arts. My teacher used to say "To be better at martial arts, all you have to do is show up." Show up on a regular basis – no matter the task – and you will most certainly improve at some point.

Fifty percent of healing can come from the acknowledgments and realisations we have. You're already half way there once you unlock your subconscious thought patterns through 'stilling your mind'. You can then start to love yourself - and forgive yourself for thinking any negative thoughts and create new ones. Some people call this the 'Law of Attraction', which came to prominence in the bestselling book *The Secret*. Others call it 'manifestation through setting intentions'. When you set intentions - and new ones that will serve you positively - the 'how' does not matter. The energy surrounding your intentions allows the universe to take care of it. In fact, the universe conspires to make it happen. All your thoughts, energy and actions start to create it. But the universe can't help you if you don't know what it is you truly want. You need to be able to say what you truly want without fear.

"Our deepest fear is not that we are inadequate. Our deepest fear is that we are powerful beyond measure. It is our light, not our darkness that most frightens us. We ask ourselves, 'Who am I to be brilliant, gorgeous, talented, fabulous?' Actually, who are you not to be? You are a child of God. Your playing small does not serve the world. There is nothing enlightened about shrinking so that other people won't feel insecure around you. We are all meant to shine, as children do. We were born to make manifest the glory of God that is within us. It's not just in some of us; it's in everyone. And as we let our own light shine, we unconsciously give other people permission to do the same. As we are liberated from our own fear, our presence automatically liberates others."[1]

This quote by author Marianne Williamson is so profound Nelson Mandela used it in one of his most memorable speeches. It also shows you why you should know yourself first and this can be discovered through the quietening of the mind. Only then can you learn to love yourself and decide you deserve it.Let your let shine so that you can give others permission to do the same.

When we set intentions for our future they are usually very specific. You may have called them 'goals' before but intentions differ slightly. Aligning your intentions in synchronicity with the lunar cycle has been practiced for centuries by people all over the world. Set your intentions by the light of a full moon to increase their power. Set yours with love over fear and try to lose any attachment to the form you think they should take. For example, your intention may be you want to create a loving family. For many people the traditional form is to get married and have two children. Try to lose attachment to this structured idea of family. There are so many different forms a family can take; there are other ways of 'feeling' married without being married; there are other ways in which to create love and unity.

be open to all the **possibilities**

Under the Tuscan Sun is a beautiful movie that illustrates this point wonderfully. The main character emerges from divorce, grieving the loss of her family. She runs away to Tuscany, Italy and tries to find herself. In doing this, she creates a community of friends. The final scene ends with her surrounded by this new community and realises she has created her own family and has all she needs. It is just in a different form to what she was previously 'attached' to. This family consists of her neighbours, gay best friend and many others. She created what I call "framily" - friends who become family too.

American talk show host Oprah Winfrey has been known to have set intentions using a ' vision board'. Bestselling author, mentor and coach, Jack Canfield, is also a fan of vision boards. He says:

"Your brain will work tirelessly to achieve the statements you give your subconscious mind. And when those statements are the affirmations and images of your goals, you are destined to achieve them!" [2]

Creating a vision board is probably one of the most valuable visualisation tools available to you. This powerful tool serves as your image of the future - a tangible representation of where you are going. Your dreams, your goals and your ideal life are all right there in front of you. As your mind responds strongly to visual stimulation, using pictures to represent your intentions will strengthen and stimulate your emotions. Your emotions are the vibrational energy that activates the 'Law of Attraction'. The saying "A picture is worth a thousand words" certainly holds true here!

How to create a **VISION BOARD** depicting the future you wish

Find pictures that represent or symbolise the experiences, feelings and possessions you want to attract into your life, and place them in your board. Have fun with the process! Use photographs, magazine cut-outs, pictures from the Internet - whatever inspires you. Be creative. Include not only pictures, but anything that speaks to you.

Consider including a picture of yourself in your board. If you do, choose one that was taken in a happy moment. You will also want to post your affirmations, inspirational words, quotations and thoughts here. Choose words and images that inspire you and make you feel good. Use only the words and images that best represent your purpose. There is beauty in simplicity and clarity. Too many images and too much information will be distracting and harder to focus on.

You can use your vision board to depict goals and dreams in all areas of your life, or concentrate on one specific area. Keep it neat and be selective about what you place in your vision board. It's a good idea to avoid creating a cluttered or chaotic board. You don't want to attract chaos into your life.

If you are working on visualising and creating changes in many areas of your life, then you may want to use more than one vision board. You might use one for your personal goals and another for career and financial goals. You might even want to keep your career vision board at the office or on your desk as a means of inspiration and affirmation.

How to use your **VISION BOARD**

Try keeping your vision board on the nightstand next to your bed. Leave it standing in an open position as often as you are comfortable and spend time each morning and evening visualising, affirming, believing and internalising your goals. The time you spend visualising in the evening just before bed is especially powerful. The thoughts and images that are present in your mind during the last 45 minutes before going to sleep are the ones that will replay themselves repeatedly in your subconscious mind throughout the night. The thoughts and images that you begin each day with will help you to create a vibrational match for the future you desire.

As some time goes by and your dreams begin to manifest, look at those images that represent your achievements and feel gratitude for how well the 'Law of Attraction' is working in your life. Acknowledge that it is working. Don't remove the pictures or images that represent the goals you've already achieved. Achievement of the goals in your vision board are powerful visual reminders of what you have already consciously and deliberately attracted into your life.

I recommend you write down the date you created your vision board. The universe loves speed, and you will be amazed at just how quickly the 'Law of Attraction' responds to your energy, commitment and desires. Much like a time capsule, this board will document your personal journey, your dreams and your achievements for that particular year. It will become a record of your growth, awareness and expansion that you will want to keep and reflect back upon in years to come.

It's a good idea to create a new vision board each year. As you continue to grow, evolve and expand, your dreams will too. Your vision board is meant to be kept and cherished. It chronicles not only your dreams, but your growth and achievements too.

Final thoughts on using your completed **VISION BOARD**

⊕ Look at your vision board often and feel the inspiration it provides.

⊕ Hold it in your hands and really internalise the future it represents.

⊕ Read your affirmations and inspirational words aloud.

⊕ See yourself living in that manner.

⊕ Feel yourself in the future you have designed.

⊕ Believe that future is already yours.

⊕ Be grateful for the good that is already present in your life.

⊕ Acknowledge any goals you have already achieved.

⊕ Acknowledge the changes you have seen and felt.

⊛   Acknowledge the presence of God or the power of the universe in your life.

For more helpful tips about vision boards visit *www.jackcanfield.com/how-to-create-an-empowering-vision-book.*

We've covered a lot of ground so far in helping you become more connected to yourself, your community and the earth itself. But what has all got to do with a digital detox, you might ask? I'll tell you.

We know we need a break from tech. But unless we set intentions about what we want to replace that act with, we will probably just lie on the couch complaining about how we can't look at our phones, or looking at the clock and wishing away the time until we can look at our technology again. Using the time and space by 'adding' to our lives with something more meaningful and purposeful is important. If we do this, we will feel happier and our soul will be nourished, thereby removing any feelings of loss we may have had. We are now 'adding to' - as opposed to 'missing out' - when you 'turn off tech'.

But how can we TEXT or POST LESS?

Keep a hand written **DIARY**

Our lives are filled with SMS's, online posts and even blog posts on all manner of social media sites and apps about how we feel. It all goes up instantly and is there permanently for the whole world to see. Do you ever stop and think 'Would I still write this if it were on pen and paper? Do you reflect on whether your posts are just a rant, venting your feelings without true reflection? How productive are your posts to you or others? If the post was directed at someone, perhaps it didn't have the same heart or loving intention that could if your saw that person face-to-face. Granted it's not always possible due to the tyranny of distance but if that person was nearby, wouldn't it have been better to create a real life connection?

Let's say we wrote these posts, our feelings, down in a book so that we could read it back to ourselves. We take the time to reflect and make changes before we decide to publish it. We'd find our thoughts would change as they do; constantly. How we feel about something now, will change in minutes, hours or days. Ask yourself if that post could have had more purpose or have been more meaningful if you had taken the time to inwardly reflect before you jumped in with both feet.

In this digital detox journey, *Wellness Load* by changing every second social media post you feel like writing online to being one in a diary or journal. Or make it a chat with someone face-to-face or over the phone. If you feel like you have nobody to talk to and tend to reach for your device for connection, know there are communities of people out there like you. Support groups, clubs and even toll free number support lines are all out there, waiting to help you in whatever way they can.

You may find that after you have written something down in a diary, you can often feel like you have already vented and don't need to publish it to the world. Chatting in person is wonderful way to connect but when we journal, we get connected with the most important person in the world; ourselves!

In this age of fast, our balance is out of whack. But why is it so important to create a more balanced state of being? There's so much more to us than just biology and physiology; achieving wellness must incorporate the mind too. You only have to look at the works of well-known authors such as Deepak Chopra. His early books spoke of his philosophy that illness can be a result of our neurology and that we can literally think ourselves into ill health. Chopra, an endocrinologist, stepped onto icy ground within his profession when he postulated this theory. But he persevered. He said:

"The mind and emotions directly affect gene activity, and since the mind is the source of a person's lifestyle and behaviour, it directs one's biological transformations. Self-awareness holds the key to this process of self-transformation. Consciousness is invisibly reaching into the biochemistry of every moment of life. In your body, as in every cell, regulation is holistic, self-generated, self-organising, and self-directed in concert with consciousness." [3]

See more at: *www.chopra.com/ccl/you-can-transform-your-own-biology*

So here is a way to create more balance in your life and nourish your mind. Choose a time in your day and set out a schedule of when you will use technology and when you will do things to slow you down and connect. Each person will have a different time of day where that will work for them. Each person will have a different schedule too, some may be weekly or monthly. Work with your lifestyle, job and responsibilities. Be flexible and kind to yourself.

If your job means being on a device, you may like to set aside a time of the week where it is not. Your boss may be able to help you with this too as you find other ways to connect with clients, or yourself. The key is balance. Connect with you.

⊕   What do you do when you're bored?

⊕   Do you reach for that handy device?

⊕   When it lights up, do you find your connection?

Stop looking for the light and **become** it instead.

We scroll through our technological devices for 'light bulb' moments, but they are not always there. Some of them come to us when the universe decides, not necessarily when we are pushing for it. Sometimes we have to trust we have done our best for that day and put our pretty little heads to rest. Let the light find you. 'Do' you instead. Turn off the tech and go and work on you!

Here's how: Take slightly less time taking photos or selfies of yourself and expand your knowledge or service in something. This may include spending that time with a charity, offering to do something for a neighbour or a company. Broaden your skill set, or broaden your knowledge of who you are. If you are lost and do not know where to begin, then good! It is only when we are lost that we will truly find ourselves.

Stillness is a wonderful way to find yourself. Some people will do this in meditation, yoga or prayer, as we have discovered. You will find your way as long as you wander where the Wi-Fi is weak. Go and explore.

If what I've said above is too 'next level' for you, I'm then going to give you some tips to help make the *Wellness Loading* easier. You can be just as present and still by being with nature, your pets or even children. When we are with a baby or child, we are attentive to their needs.

We're forced to 'be in the moment'. I know being with an infant may be exhausting at times, but there's so much joy in so many moments too. Spending quality time with your children or even a friend's – sans your devices – is a wonderful way to *Wellness Load*.

For some, I do understand that it can be a real challenge to sit still. So besides connecting with food, nature and community, here is another way to reconnect with yourself:

create **connectedness**
through practising **gratitude** daily.

In a world where we feel we never have enough, I reflect now on how to practice the art of ratitude. First, create quiet. Even if it is only for 15 minutes a day. Your act of *Wellness Loading* does not have to be for a whole hour. Start with whatever you can do, but make it focused, concentrated and at committed time.

Practising being grateful for what you have and you will attract more. You may even recognise that you are already abundant and have a shift in perception. It may bring about a sense of peace that you never knew was possible. This is true **WELLNESS.** Then, and only then, if you are meant to have **MORE,** then you will be presented with just that.

Try this set of thoughts and actions specifically:

⊕ Remove thoughts of the past and future.

⊕ Be in the now.

⊕ Focus on your breath.

trust you have everything you need right now, and all will present itself, if the **universe** feels you need that too.

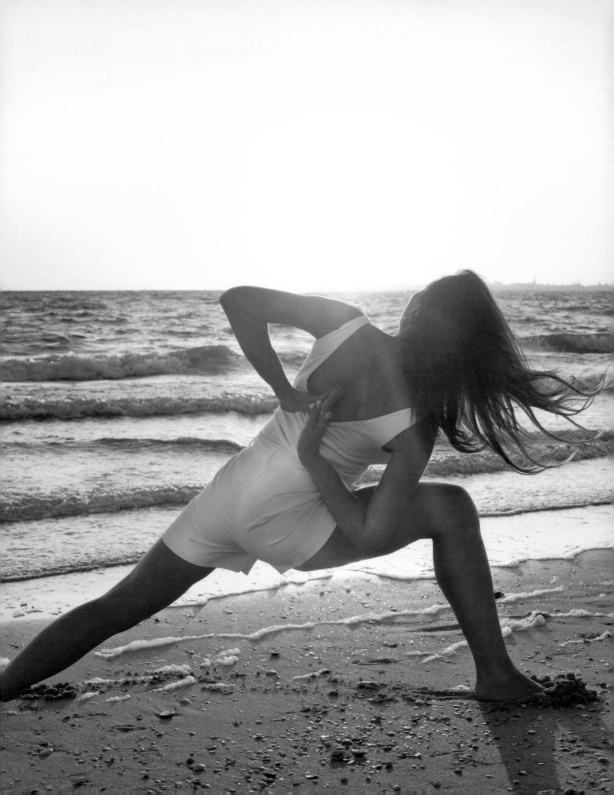

⊕ Be still.

⊕ Rest.

⊕ When your 'in' breath is the same as your 'out' breath, you will be more balanced.

Decide to do this at least once a day. It may only be for a few minutes and you may decide to extend that period of time the better you get at it. It's like building up skill or increasing your fitness. Take your time to build it up.

I have known many successful entrepreneurs who have difficulty even switching off for a few minutes. You may decide that being out in nature is going to be better for you to be able to practice the art of breathing and meditation. If this suits you better, go for it.

Other ways of switching off may be with an activity. You don't always need to be still. Some claim that whilst they are doing Tai Chi, BJJ martial arts, rock climbing, skipping, mountain trekking, walking along the beach, swimming or surfing, that they have felt at one with nature and rejuvenated.

There is one thing all of these activities have in common: the breath and being in the moment. When you swim, do Tai Chi or skip, you create a rhythm and pattern of breathing. When you are performing a martial arts manoeuvre or surfing, you need to be in that moment, so you are ready to roll with whatever comes at you; it could be another movement of attack you need to defend, or the intense focus on the roll of the waves. Which wave will you surf? When will you decide to paddle or stand? And if it doesn't go the way you had planned, how do you 'go with the flow' instead of resisting the ride of life?

I have experienced stillness of the mind recently in a floatation tank too. It was a bath of warm water, rich in magnesium that helps you to float. Your body does not sink. The feeling of weightlessness helped all my muscles to relax and let go. Often when we lie on a bed or even a massage table, our muscles are still engaged and working. Being in a floatation tank helps you to completely surrender as your muscles are totally relaxed with the water supporting you. Others like to use an infrared or steam room sauna.
Get creative with ways in which you can reconnect when you disconnect. It does not have to be one set way of meditation. Allow the form of meditation that is right for you to express

itself. There is a myriad of things you can do when you look for them. Set intentions to find what's right for you and the universe will conspire to help you find it.

decide to **seek**, and you shall find.

If you seek negativity, you will find it and attract it. If you want only peace and happiness for others, then you will be able to find that too. Your consciousness will open up to looking for the love or the good in all things. You will be able to attract and create that because we are all only reflections of each other.

find your **soul purpose.**

When we have the courage to admit what we really love and pursue that is when we are truly at our happiest. Our souls sing when we are talk about our passions. Have you ever watched a very talented person and been blown away by them? A person delivering a presentation, a singer on stage, an artist in his zone, a musician, doctor in their element, or a parent nurturing naturally. It is certainly an attractive quality. Sometimes I call it a 'talent crush'. We are drawn to the beauty of their truth but more so, their **AUTHENTICITY.**

We love people who are the truth; we smell the phonies from miles away.

Have you ever been told you could never make a living doing something you love? What limiting self-belief systems do you have? Who told you the lie? Dr John Demartini, healer, speaker, philosopher, author, chiropractor and contributor to bestseller *The Secret* was told because he was dyslexic, he would amount to nothing. He used this as motivation to teach himself to read and literally had a truck load of books delivered to his door. He studied how to become a speed reader and read everything he could about the jaw, an area of the body he'd always been interested in. He then started teaching orthodontists, sharing his findings, which then led him to becoming a chiropractor so he could study the rest of the body. Amazing.

Step up and have the courage to now admit what you truly yearn to do. Courage comes from the French word *le couer* which means heart. To have courage is to have heart. And the heart is never wrong. This, my friend, is your soul purpose. And as I type that, I type it with gratitude in my heart. For it was Dr John Demartini who taught me this in his *Breakthrough Experience* program and put me on the path to live my inspired life. He wrote the foreword to my first book and you're now reading my sixth! I am now compelled to pay it forward to you.

When you find the courage to admit what you love and do it is when you will feel a sense of peace and calm. You've found your soul purpose. You have *Wellness Loaded.* You are what I term as **BEING ON PATH** and you won't need to check your device so often. This is what I want for you, because I know you do too.

I too, suffer from device addiction and we all do at some point. But we need to address the cause, not just the symptom. I can tell you "Get rid of your phone for the day!" and you may do it for the day because I told you so. But how long will this last? That's why I believe you will be more inspired to implement periods of reconnection and acts of wellness when you feel like you have done things for **YOURSELF,** all by yourself and not just because someone told you that you should.

This is why wellness coaching works. It helps people to build their self-efficacy and self-confidence, so much so that they are able to make their own life decisions, for a better lifestyle and for the long term. Figure out your soul purpose, work that into your lifestyle. Have the confidence to ask.

It's very easy for me to say 'have self-confidence' but developing it can be a lifelong work-in-progress. All confidence though is having trust. Therefore, you might need to work on your **TRUST MUSCLE.**

- ➲ How do you trust?
- ➲ So many fears come into play like what if I fail?
- ➲ What if they don't like me?

I could continue sharing examples for quite some time. But from an NLP perspective, (neuro-linguistic programming), how about we try to re-program your brain with what it really needs.

- ➲ Are you ready?
- ➲ What if you are exactly where you need to be?
- ➲ What if you need to 'learn the lessons'?

Release the part of you that needs to know 'why' and focus on the spiritual lesson for growth. My martial arts training taught me there no winning and losing, only winning and learning. In which case, you are always winning aren't you? If losing is imperative for growth, then sit in that 'divine discomfort' and know that it too shall pass, because you will be richer in lessons through another life experience.

Now that you know this, you can

trust the journey.
hold your **vision** close and **trust the process.**

When you put this perspective into practice on a daily basis, you may find that a lot of anxiety or attention span difficulties may subside. Boom! You may have just removed some of the cause of why you are so addicted to your device!

You are now ready to begin your choices of daily *Wellness Loading.*

Enjoy the reconnected MINDFUL RECIPES and WELLNESS LOADING JOURNAL that are contained in the following pages.

RECIPES

CHAPTER FIVE

Nurture via nature with these Mindful Food recipes. Eating as close to nature as possible helps you keep reconnected and promotes wellbeing.

Terms: tsp = teaspoon tbs = tablespoon

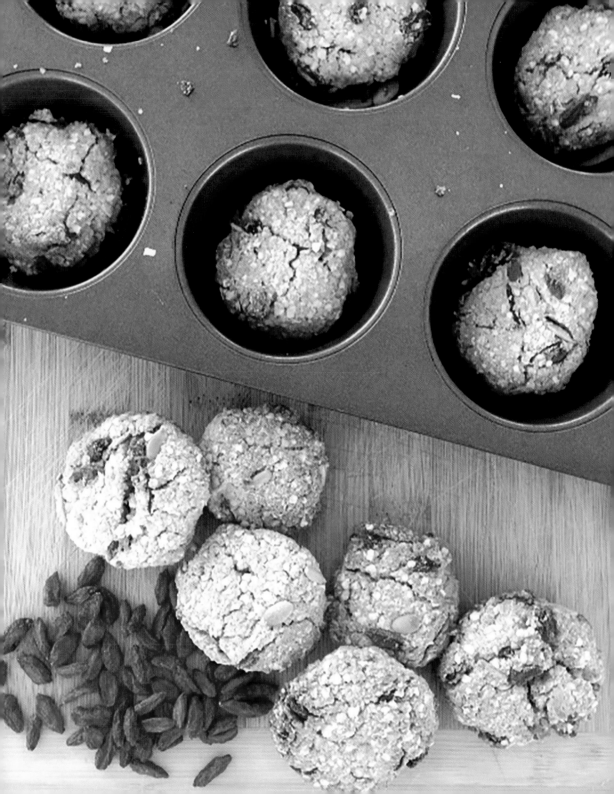

GOJI BERRY COOKIES TO GO!

12 small cookies

Ingredients

½ cup desiccated coconut

2 tbs pepitas and sunflower seeds

2 tbs almond meal

2 tbs RAW vegan Amazonia protein powder

2 cup rolled quinoa flakes

2 tbs goji berries

1 tsp vanilla essence

2 tbs organic peanut butter

2 tbs organic rice malt syrup or coconut flower nectar

2 tbs butter

2 tbs coconut oil - slightly solidified

Method

Preheat oven to 180 degrees Celsius.

Add all ingredients to a bowl and mix with hands until sticky when pressed between the fingers. Add a little bit more sweetener if the mixture does not stick together.

Line a baking tray or use a non-stick muffin tray.

Scoop 1 tbsp of the cookie mixture, roll into balls and firmly press almond into the cookie dough to sit in each hole of the muffin tray.

Bake in the oven for approximately 30-45 mins.

Keep the cookies in an airtight container.

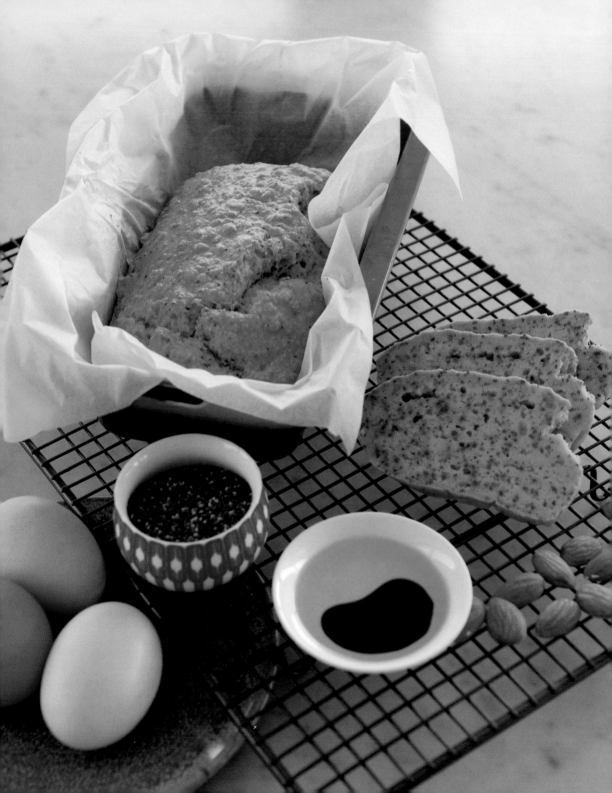

PALEO BREAD

Serves 3 - 4

Ingredients

¾ cup of rice flour or quinoa flour
or coconut flour

1 cup almond meal

2 tbs chia seeds

3 free-range, organic and hormone-free eggs

2 tbs apple cider vinegar

1 tbs baking powder

Pinch of pink Peruvian salt

1 cup of water

Method

Pre-heat oven 175 degrees Celsius.

Sift flour and almond meal into a bowl, soak chia seeds in a half a cup of water for a few minutes. Add gel-like chia seeds, eggs and the rest of ingredients and mix.

Pour into a baking paper lined small loaf tin. Bake in oven for 25 - 30 mins.

Serve with olive oil and Jomeis organic sweet reduction balsamic vinegar, organic butter or coconut butter.

Also you could eat with organic peanut butter for extra fat and protein. Other good fat spreads are things like goats cheese or avocado and healthy cacao chocolate spreads.

For kids' parties, find additive and colouring free sprinkles from your local health foods shop to create the fairy bread bites.

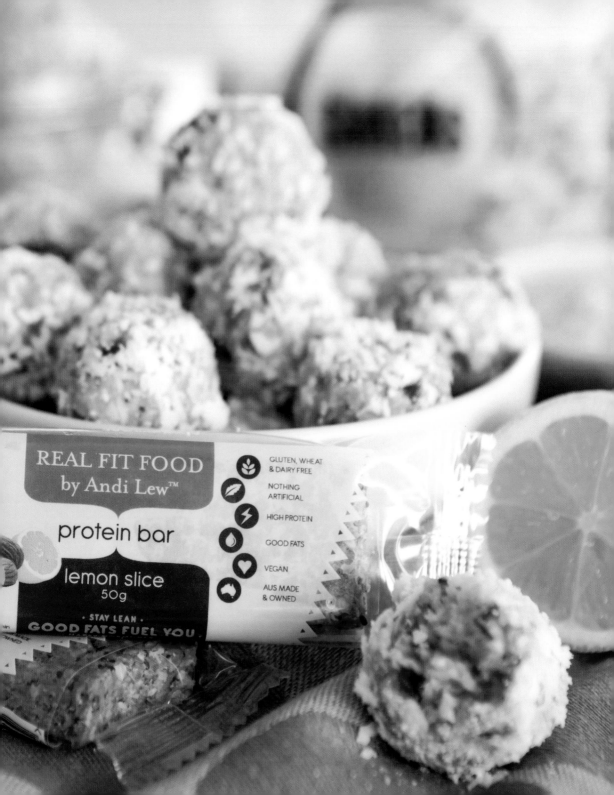

REAL FIT FOOD
by Andi Lew™

protein bar

lemon slice
50g

· STAY LEAN ·
GOOD FATS FUEL YOU

GLUTEN, WHEAT
& DAIRY FREE

NOTHING
ARTIFICIAL

HIGH PROTEIN

GOOD FATS

VEGAN

AUS MADE
& OWNED

LIMONCELLO SUPERFOOD PROTEIN BOMBS

Makes 15-20 balls

Ingredients

3 cups almond meal

½ cup shredded coconut

½ cup solidified coconut oil (if the oil is liquid, it will still work, but you just need to solidify the balls in the fridge once rolled)

6 pitted medjool dates

Rind of 2 lemons

3 tbsp Amazonia Raw pea protein isolate - plain or vanilla

½ cup chia seeds, soaked in ½ cup water

Method

Throw all ingredients in a food processor, then roll into balls. You may need to add a little water to help bind it. Then roll, and cover in desiccated coconut.

Keep in the fridge and let it set.

Eat straight from the fridge because coconut oil solidifies when it's cold and becomes an oil when it's hot. Have with a cup of peppermint tea!

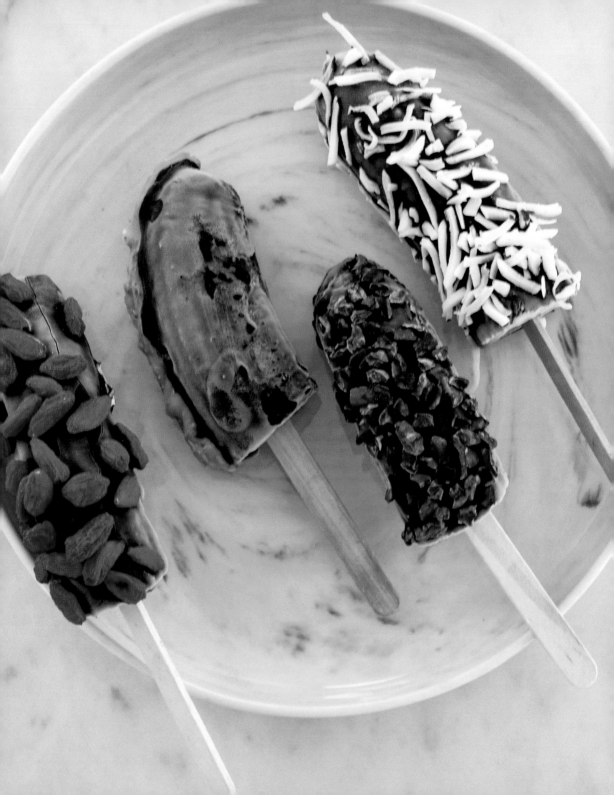

BANANA POPS

Makes 8

Ingredients

4 bananas

8 popsicle sticks

1 block of dark, sugar free chocolate (there are many brands in health stores that are sweetened with rice malt syrup, agave nectar and use coconut oil with cacao)

Superfoods for coating - chia seeds, coconut flakes, cacao nibs, crunchy peanut butter

Method

Place chocolate in a metal bowl and sit bowl over a saucepan filled with hot simmering water. Be careful to constantly stir until melted and do not allow any water to find its way into the bowl or the chocolate will seize.

After the chocolate is melted, coat your bananas with it, adding any Superfoods along with it. Put in the freezer to solidify banana and coating. Eat in about 2 hours.

* You can also make your own vegan/dairy free chocolate by melting:

1 cup coconut oil

1 cacao butter nugget - optional

2 heaped tbs cacao powder

2-3 tbs of coconut syrup or rice malt syrup for a lower GI version

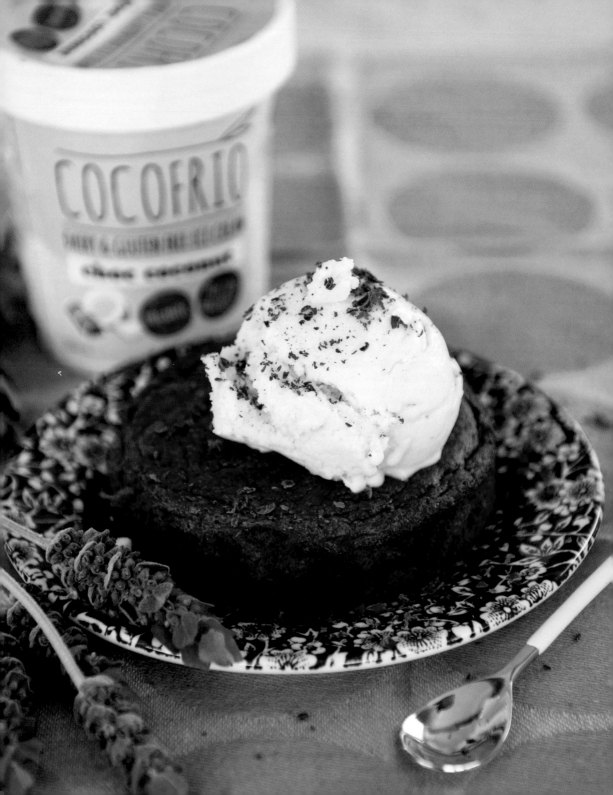

PALEO CHOCOLATE CAKE

Serves 2-4

You won't believe this cake actually contains no dairy, no gluten, no flour, no sugar and no wheat! It's the cake, that's not cake! Make sure your kids finish all the cake before they leave the table.

Ingredients

100g sugar and dairy free dark chocolate

1 teaspoon vanilla extract

2 overripe bananas

½ cup roasted or boiled sweet potato

¼ cup honey or ½ cup rice malt syrup

1 whole egg, free-range, organic and hormone-free

3 egg whites, free-range, organic and hormone-free

Method

Preheat oven to 200 degrees Celsius.

Place 8 custard cups or 2 small cake spring tins on a large baking sheet. Line with baking paper or coconut oil or butter and set aside.

Combine chocolate and vanilla extract in a medium bowl over hot boiling water. Whisk until chocolate is completely melted. Be careful not to let it burn as it will melt quickly.

Puree bananas, boiled sweet potato and honey until smooth.

Remove the melted chocolate from heat and fold it over banana puree and egg. The folding technique, used with a cake spatula, helps to keep the cake mixture aerated. Mix well.

In a separate bowl, whip the egg whites until soft peaks form. Slowly fold egg whites into chocolate mixture. Keep it aerated.

Spoon mixture into ramekins, filling them almost to the top.

Bake for approximately 6-7 minutes, remove and serve. The centre of each cake should be soft and warm. Garnish with fresh cream if you like, or a coconut yogurt or COCOFRIO coconut ice-cream for a dairy free option.

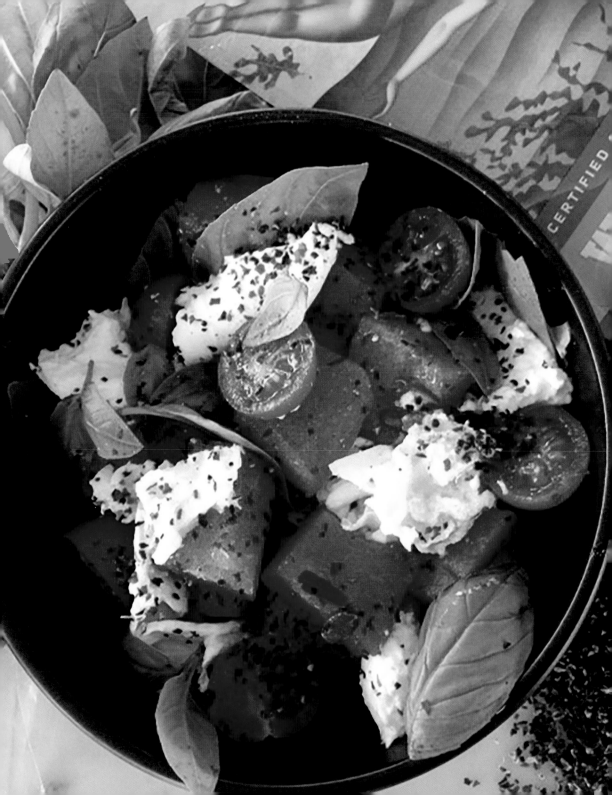

WATERMELON SALAD

Serves 2-4

Ingredients

½ watermelon cut into cubes

1 punnet of cherry tomatoes halved

½ bunch of fresh basil leaves

1 buffalo mozzarella ball

Salts of the Earth - pink varieties

Crushed seaweed/nori (optional)

2 tbs cold pressed organic olive oil

Method

Combine all ingredients in the following order; the watermelon cubes and tomatoes first, then tear the cheese and basil leaves on top. Try not to mix this salad too much to avoid the watermelon cubes from changing shape.

Serve immediately.

This salad is best eaten straight away and not stored, as it can become watery/soggy if eaten the next day.

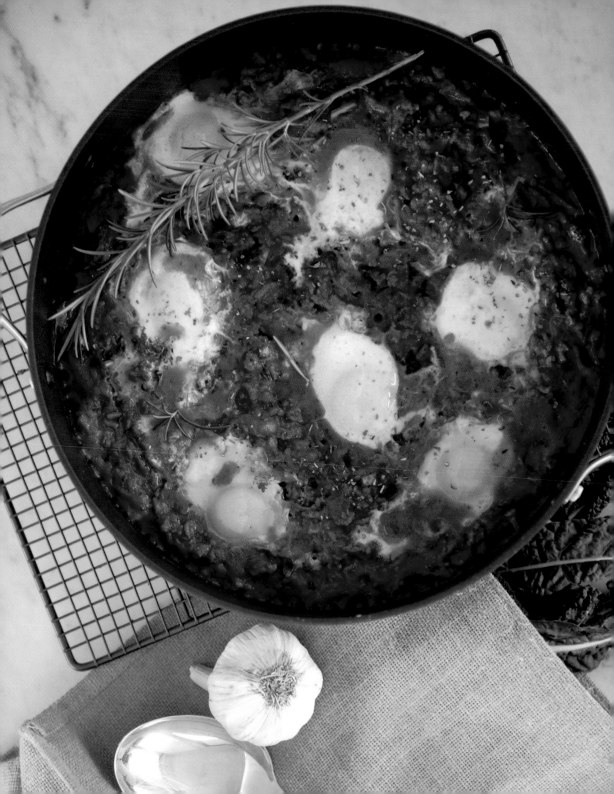

ISRAELI SHAKSHUKA

Serves 2

Ingredients

1 jar or 4 tbs concentrated tomato paste

1 can or bottle of tomato puree

Boiled cauliflower pieces

Handful of washed spinach leaves

2 cloves of crushed garlic

½ diced brown onion

1 tbs paprika

4 free-range, organic and hormone-free eggs

Superfoods pink salt to taste

Crushed black pepper corns

Coconut oil for frying

Method

Fry onion and garlic in oil in a shallow pan until slightly browned.

Add cauliflower and continue to fry for about two minutes.

Add the crushed tomato puree and paste to the mix. Stir well, heating it up on a low heat.

Add the spices and wilt the spinach leaves through. You now have a tomato pasta base.

Make a space to cook 4 eggs. Crack eggs and continue to let fry on a low heat with a lid on the pan.

Eat straight away and serve with Paleo bread or rye toast!

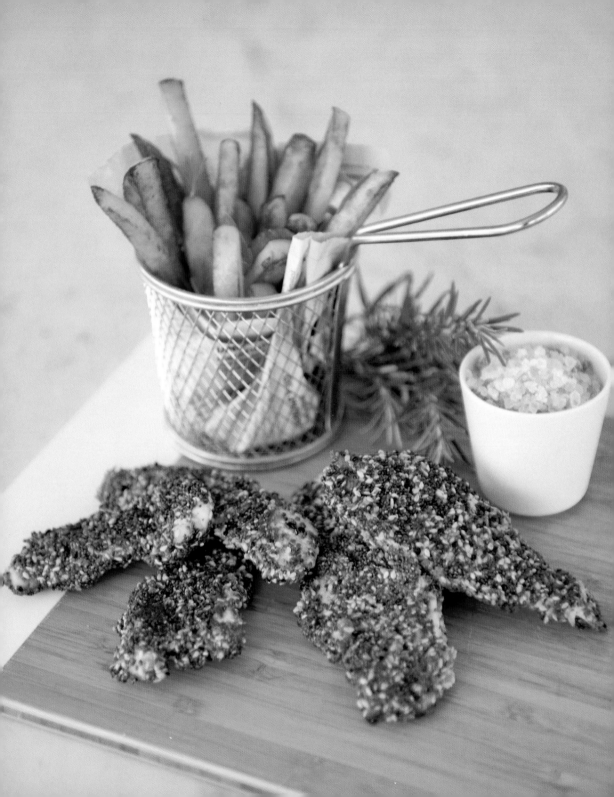

GLUTEN-FREE
SUPER SEED CRUMBED CHICKEN

Serves 4

Ingredients

4 organic, free-range and hormone free chicken breast fillets

2 organic, free-range and hormone-free eggs

½ cup rice crumbs or tapioca flour

½ cup sesame seeds

¼ cup chia seeds

2 tbs cumin powder

Superfoods pink salt

Coconut oil for frying

Method

Slice the chicken breast in the middle so you have halved the thickness. The thinner the pieces, the easier it is to ensure it's cooked all the way through.

Prepare two shallow bowls, one with raw eggs beaten and the other with the dry ingredients.

Coat and dip the chicken in the eggs, then dip into the mixed dry ingredients. Use tongs because the coating can stick to your fingers. Shallow fry in oil. Try not to turn over too often. Make sure the chicken is well browned before you flip it to ensure it's cooked all the way through.

Serve with Israeli purple salad and a tahini sauce. Serve with mindful fries (see next recipe).

MINDFUL FRIES

These are the fries that are actually safe and good for you! Most of us avoid eating deep fried foods because they're carcinogenic (cancer causing). It's the trans-fats that we should avoid but frying in coconut oil solves this problem. It is the only oil that doesn't denature, or lose its molecular structure when you heat it past a certain temperature. Frying any food in coconut oil is safe. Using other oil turns it into a trans-fat.

I often make these for my son as a treat. Boys need three times the amount of carbohydrates than girls. Some often get a craving for salty foods. Chips or fries are usually on the top of this list. If you notice that you're craving salt, you could be deficient in magnesium. Salts of the Earth is the good kind in the real food form and totally unprocessed. It is rich in minerals like magnesium. It is the processed version of salt we must avoid. This is called iodised salt.

If you are craving salt, you may also be dehydrated. Salt helps attract and retain water. So if you are needing more water in your body, you will often crave salt. The best thing to do is go back to rehydrating with real, live foods that are full of water, and drink alkalized water. Then start to include magnesium rich foods like dark leafy greens, cacao and pink salts.

Ingredients

5 large potatoes

Coconut oil

Pink Salts of the Earth

Method

Peel and chop potatoes into medium or thin shaped fries. Shallow fry in a pan with coconut oil. Serve with pink Salts of the Earth.

Use a home-made organic tomato sauce if possible. Most tomato sauce brands are sugar-laden.

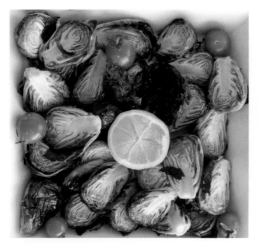

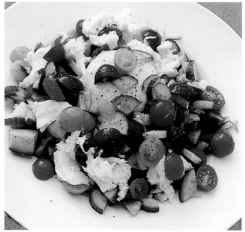

BRUSSEL SPROUT CHIPS

Serves 4

Ingredients
Half a tbs pink Peruvian salt

About 12-20 Brussel sprouts

Olive oil

Method

Cut all Brussel sprouts in half and place on a lined baking tray. Sprinkle with salt and drizzle with oil.

Place in an oven set to 180 degrees Celsius for about 30/40 mins or until golden and crunchy on the outside and 'softish' on the inside.

Serve with lemon wedges and cherry tomatoes.

Add more Superfoods salt to taste for extra magnesium. Yum!

MINDFUL MEDITERRANEAN SALAD

Serves 4

Ingredients
1 punnet of multi-coloured cherry tomatoes

2 Lebanese cucumbers

1 mozzarella ball or some cubes of sheep's or goat's milk feta

Handful of marinated black pitted olives

Salts of the Earth pink salt

Ground black peppercorns

Cold pressed virgin organic olive oil

½ Spanish/purple onion

Method

Cube all vegetables and crumble/tear cheese through the salad. Add other ingredients to taste. Tomatoes are very rich in antioxidants and the olives and olive oil are a helpful anti-ageing food as they're full of lots of good fats our hormones and nerve system need.

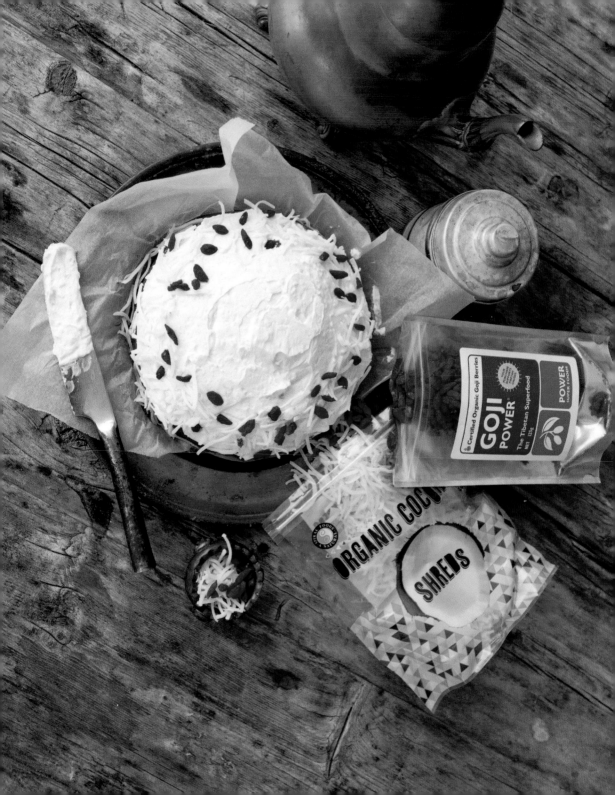

CREAMY COCONUT CARROT CAKE

Serves 10-12

Ingredients

2 cups self-raising spelt, rice or tapioca flour. If you can't get self-raising flour, then add 2 tbs baking powder to your gluten-free flour

1 tsp ground cinnamon

1 cup xylitol

2 cups grated carrots

1 cup chopped walnuts

4 free-range, organic and hormone-free eggs, lightly beaten

2 cups coconut oil

Topping

1 cup goat's cream cheese

Juice of 1 lemon

½ cup xylitol/stevia powder (be careful the brand you choose isn't bitter. Some will be blended with fruit sugars to make it less bitter)

Walnuts, shredded coconut and goji berries to top and garnish

Method

Pre-heat oven to 180 - 160°C fan forced. Grease a 6cm deep, 19cm square tin or medium round tin with coconut oil. Line base and sides with baking paper.

Sift flour and cinnamon into a bowl. Add xylitol, carrots, chopped walnuts, coconut oil and eggs. Stir to combine.

Spread into prepared tin. Bake for 1 hour and 15 minutes or until a skewer inserted comes out clean. Cover loosely with foil or baking paper if it is over-browning too quickly. Stand in pan for 10 minutes. Turn out onto a wire rack to cool.

Once cooled, prepare frosting by blending the cream cheese, lemon and stevia or xylitol with a beater on a low speed. Spread over cake. Add all garnishes and serve.

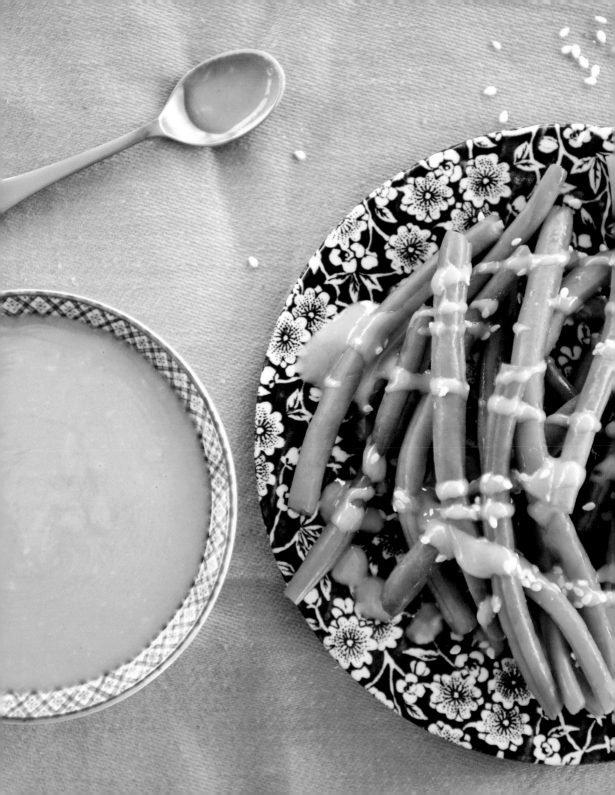

SWEET HALVA TAHINI DRESSING

Serves 6-10

Ingredients

½ jar of Spiral Foods hulled tahini (the lighter coloured one)

Pink Peruvian sea salt

1 large clove of crushed garlic

½ cup Jomeis organic sweet reduction balsamic vinegar

½ cup olive or flaxseed oil

¼ cup Spiral Foods organic apple cider vinegar

Method

Empty half the jar of tahini into a food processor and add all other ingredients. Blend until creamy.

Drizzle over any vegetables, like steamed greens and sprinkle with sesame seeds.

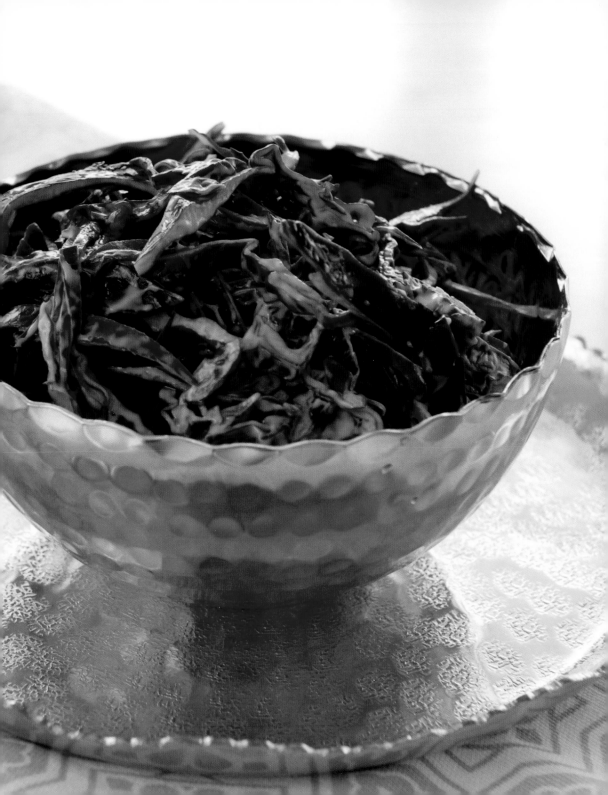

PURPLE ISRAELI CABBAGE SALAD

Serves 2-4

Ingredients

½ purple cabbage

1 large garlic crushed clove

Superfoods pink salt to taste

Juice of half a lemon

2 heaped tbs of sugar free mayonnaise

Method

Shred/cut the cabbage into fine slices.

Add the rest of the ingredients and mix very well until it softens a little.

Transfer to a cleaner bowl (because it can dirty the plate with purple colour).

This salad always tastes better the next day as it ferments a little. It can last in an airtight container for a few days.

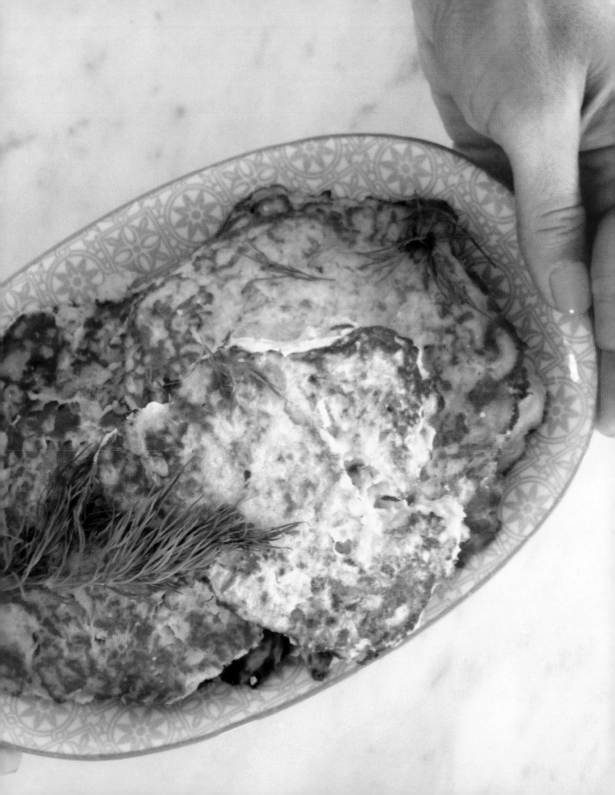

PALEO ZUCCHINI FRITTERS

Makes 6-8

Ingredients

6 free-range, organic and hormone-free eggs

1 cup coconut flour

Salt

½ cup nut milk

2 large grated zucchinis

1 brown grated onionw

Coconut oil for frying

Method

Combine all ingredients, except the oil into a bowl and mix until you get a pancake batter.

Fry in a pan on medium heat like you would a pancake.

Serve with dill, mayonnaise and fried, poached or boiled eggs or greens!

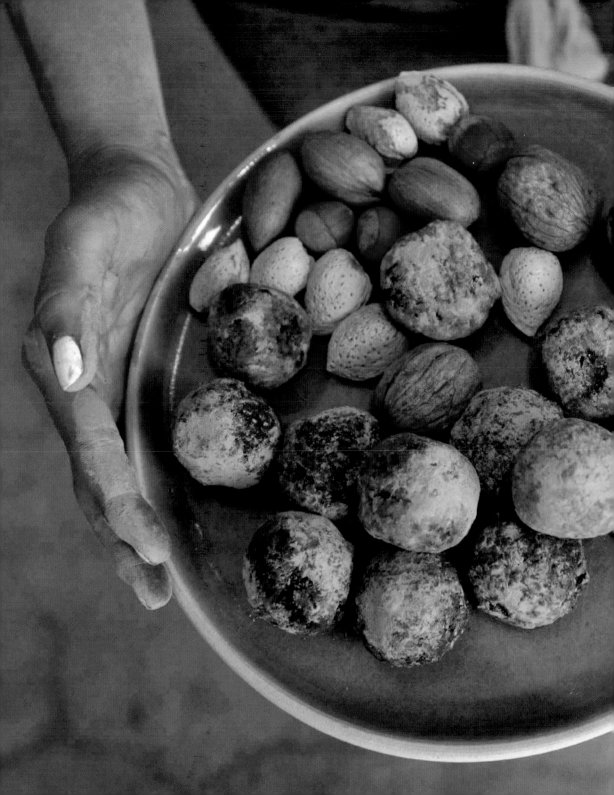

GREEN TEA AMAZEBALLS

Makes 15 balls

Ingredients

2 cups quinoa oat flakes (gluten-free options), or rolled oats

1 cup pitted dates, roughly chopped

½ cup of shredded coconut

½ cup of sultanas

½ cup of almonds

2 tbs organic peanut butter

1 tbs cocoa powder

2 tbs honey

¾ tbs or more filtered and alkalized water

1 tsp vanilla extract

Organic green tea powder for rich antioxidants and metabolism booster

Method

Put all ingredients apart from the water and green tea powder into a food processor and blend until it has the consistency of breadcrumbs. Add the water and continue to process until it becomes sticky enough to roll into balls.

Use a tablespoon to measure the mixture and roll into firm balls. Roll into green tea powder to make the outside look pretty and store in an airtight container in the fridge.

<u>Note:</u> You'll need to make sure the peanut butter is a good quality, pesticide-free kind. Spiral Foods do a great one. If you're concerned about nut allergies, you can use a different type of nut butter or cold-pressed organic coconut oil instead.

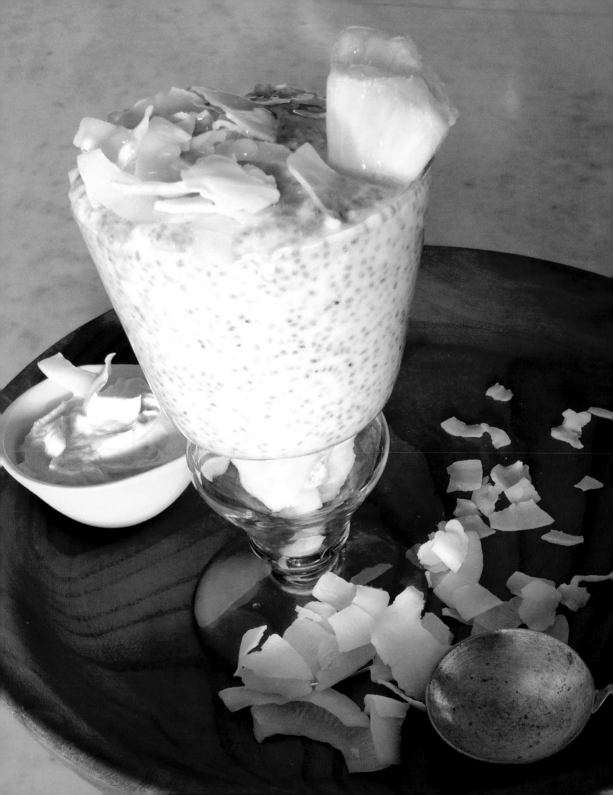

CHIA COLADA

Serves 2-4

A modern wellness spin on Pina Colada, this dessert, snack or breakfast has the taste of the islands with coconut and pineapple, and is packed with micro-nutrition (vitamins and minerals) and loaded with Superfoods and good fats.

Ingredients

3 cups of chia seeds

2 cans of coconut cream, not low-fat milk

Sweetening options

3 tbs rice malt syrup or 2tbs coconut syrup or honey

1 tsp pure vanilla essence

Top with pineapple and coconut flakes or shreds

Method

Place chia seeds and coconut cream into a bowl and stir constantly. The chia seeds like to absorb liquid and will continue to expand and absorb over a period of 5 minutes or more. Once thick, like a pudding, add sweetener and vanilla essence.

Then serve in a glass, jar or bowl and top with fruit and flakes.

Variations: add passionfruit and banana.

Serve and eat immediately. It can be stored, but keep in mind, once in the fridge, it will become harder set and less creamy. Since it only takes a few minutes to make, this dish is best made and enjoyed right away!

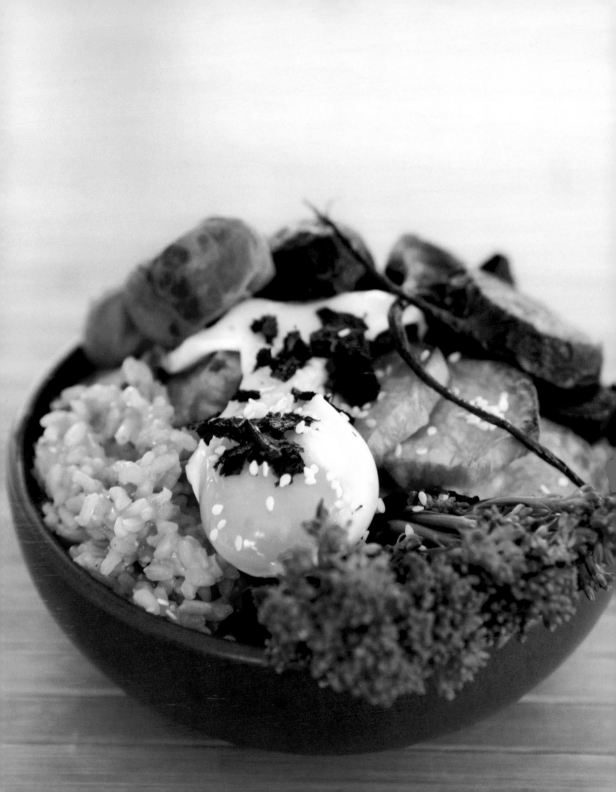

MACRO BOWL

Serves 1-2

Ingredients

2 cups brown rice

1 tbs miso paste

1 cup broccoli

½ small sweet potato

2 kimchee fermented Japanese plums

1 soft boiled free-range, organic and hormone-free egg

Sesame seeds

Japanese Superfood Wakeme or Nori flakes

3 baby beets

Olive oil or coconut oil

Pink Salts of the Earth

Method

Prepare the rice by boiling in a pan with 3 cups of water to 2 cups of rice. Brown rice takes a little longer to cook than white rice, so you may need to monitor and add more water.

Set aside and once cooled slightly, add the miso paste and stir through with salt to taste.

Roast the veggies with the oil and salt. Set aside and prepare the soft boiled egg.

Place the rice in a bowl and add roasted vegetables and boiled egg.

Garnish with black or white sesame seeds and the Wakame or Nori flakes.

Eat right away!

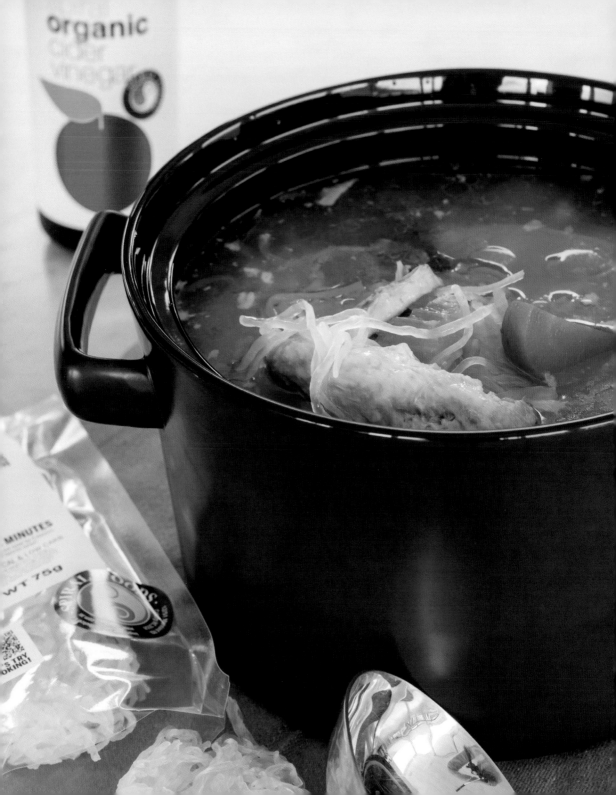

GUT HEALING BONE BROTH

Serves 6

This is what we used to call 'Jewish Penicillin' because of the healing properties the broth gives to the gut. Organic apple cider vinegar helps draw out collagen from the bones of the bird, and collagen repairs tissue. Bone broth helps to repair the lining of the stomach wall. This is perfect if you have leaky gut syndrome or have had an overuse of medication recently. I use the Spiral Foods brand of vinegar. Please DO NOT forget the key ingredient when making this chicken broth! Also, make sure the chicken you use has had no added hormones, is organic and was free to roam.

Ingredients

Whole organic, free-range, hormone free chicken

½ cup Spiral Foods Organic apple cider vinegar

2 celery sticks

2 carrots

½ pot alkalized water

1 bay leaf

Pink Salts of the Earth

Method

Put the whole bird in a pressure cooker or slow cooker, and fill with alkalized water until the bird is covered.

Add the rest of the ingredients and cook for at least 4-8 hours.

Drink often, and even in the mornings instead of coffee.

Serve with buckwheat noodles or shitake noodles.

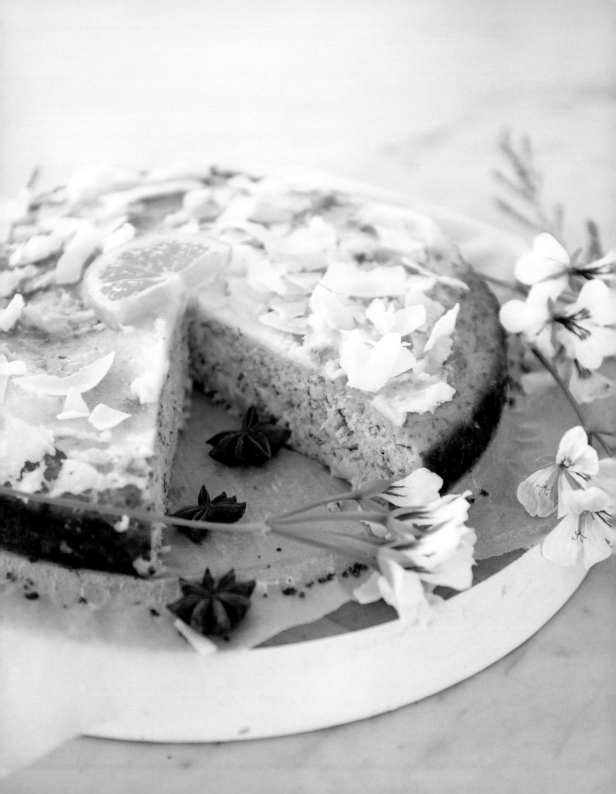

LEMON AND CHIA SEED CAKE

Serves 12

Ingredients

3 lemons - tops removed/cut
and scored with a cross about 3cm deep

6 free-range, organic and hormone-free eggs

200g xylitol

250g almond meal

3 tsp baking powder

5 tbs chia seeds soaked in a cup of water

Method

I know the 'lemon' prep sounds time-consuming - and it is! – but please try it. Once you've prepped them, the mixing time is very quick and you'll be done before you know it!

Prep your lemons. Then place the prepared lemons in boiling water and simmer for 50 minutes. Remove from the water and purée the whole lemons, including peel in a food processor, until smooth.

Preheat the oven to 160 degrees Celsius.

In a large mixing bowl, mix the eggs and xylitol until light and fluffy. Add the almond meal and baking powder. Mix until combined. Stir in the lemon purée and soaked chia seeds. Pour the mixture into a 22cm cake tin lined with greaseproof baking paper. Spring tins are best so that the cake doesn't stick to the bottom and sides. Do not use foil. Bake in the oven for 40 minutes or until firm but still moist. It may need to cook for up to 50 minutes. Leave to cool in the tin for about 5 minutes then turn onto a wire rack.

Topping: Blend solidified cold pressed coconut oil with xylitol or coconut sugar to taste. Sprinkle coconut chips on top. Keep cool so that the coconut oil doesn't liquify.

Note: This cake is a really wet cake and can stay fresh for a few days. It can be served warm with sheep's milk yoghurt or Cocofrio Ice-cream, dolloped on the side. The almond meal provides a gluten-free treat and is high in protein. This is a twist on the traditional orange and poppy seed cake, but the chia seeds are very high in essential fatty acids. It's a great way of consuming chia seeds.

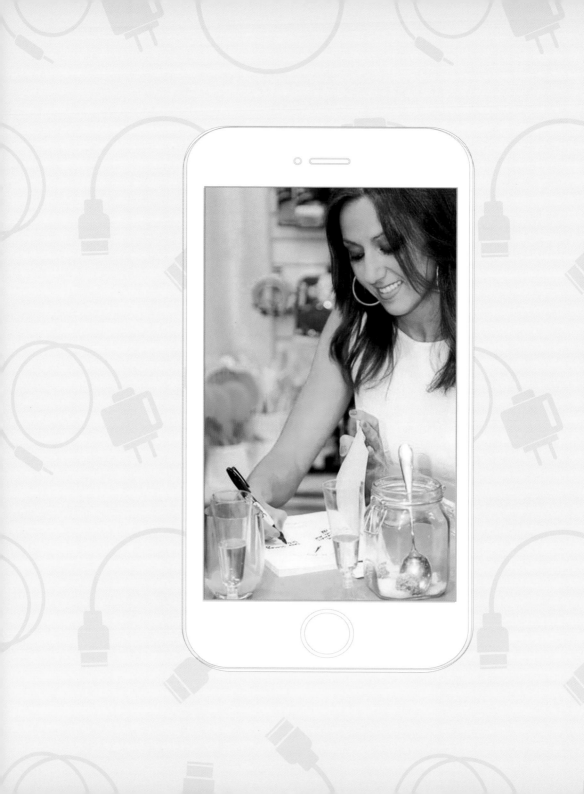

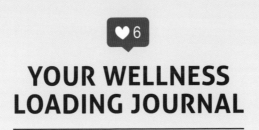

YOUR WELLNESS
LOADING JOURNAL

CHAPTER SIX

"When asked what gift he wanted for his birthday, the yogi
replied: I wish no gifts, only presence." ~ Unknown

YOUR JOURNALLING SPACE is a place where you can keep a record of your thoughts and feelings and reflect upon them - instead of posting or texting. You may still decide to publish them but it will be after reflection and be from a more balanced perspective.

Your *Wellness Loading* Journal is the space to set out your intentions for the week.

Mark down each day with five things you have chosen to do to create more connectedness. If you decide to do something that reconnects you more than five days a week, then there is the space for that too.

Here are some choices:

- 10 second hugs

- Eating more plants/less meat

- Nourishing your body and soul by cooking at home

- Filling your love tank and doing something kind for you

- Fitness or some sort of physical movement/activity

- Practising gratitude

- Paying it forward/acts of service

- Hydrating with alkalized water

- Turning off tech one hour before sleep

- Going to sleep with the natural Lunar cycle

- Taking time to practice slow and connected breathing

⊛   Shopping for real, whole foods at a farmer's market

⊛   Nurturing your soul by being with nature

⊛   Writing hand written letters of gratitude

⊛   Practising yoga

⊛   Culling your clutter and donating it to those in need

These are just suggestions but feel free to come up with your own thoughts and acts of *Wellness Loading.* I hope the previous pages have inspired you to do so.

An example of a *Wellness Loading* Journal could look like this:

MONDAY

THOUGHTS - I chose this day of the week to reconnect by preparing food at home. Monday was the day I was born and I find it to be my most productive day of the week, so I want to detox from tech when I get home from work and cook with my son.

TO SHARE THESE FEELINGS WITH - During this experience I discovered ... and I decided to share these feelings with .... OR I decided to keep them to myself.

I also decided to go to sleep at 10pm and turned off my technology an hour prior. Instead, I read and played music. I know I have a big work meeting and a couple of parties later this week, so I decided to start with a big day of Wellness Loading today to balance out the fun and late nights I plan to have later.

🏠 Home   ♡ Share   ☁ Add to Shortcuts   ☆ Favourites   ⏱ Timeout

---

MONDAY

⌂ Home   ♡ Share   ☁ Add to Shortcuts   ☆ Favourites   ⏰ Timeout

TUESDAY

⌂ Home   ♡ Share   ☁ Add to Shortcuts   ☆ Favourites   ⏰ Timeout

WEDNESDAY

....

....

....

....

....

....

....

....

....

⌂ Home   ♡ Share   ☁ Add to Shortcuts   ☆ Favourites   ⏱ Timeout

THURSDAY

....

....

....

....

....

....

....

....

....

⌂ Home   ♡ Share   ☁ Add to Shortcuts   ☆ Favourites   ⏱ Timeout

FRIDAY

....

....

....

....

....

....

....

....

⌂ Home　♡ Share　☁ Add to Shortcuts　☆ Favourites　⏱ Timeout

SATURDAY

....

....

....

....

....

....

....

....

⌂ Home　♡ Share　☁ Add to Shortcuts　☆ Favourites　⏱ Timeout

SUNDAY

⌂ Home   ♡ Share   ☁ Add to Shortcuts   ☆ Favourites   ⏰ Timeout

NOTES: A WEEK OF REFLECTIONS

MONDAY

⌂ Home ♡ Share ☁ Add to Shortcuts ☆ Favourites ⏱ Timeout

TUESDAY

⌂ Home ♡ Share ☁ Add to Shortcuts ☆ Favourites ⏱ Timeout

WEDNESDAY

⌂ Home   ♡ Share   ☁ Add to Shortcuts   ☆ Favourites   ⏲ Timeout

THURSDAY

⌂ Home   ♡ Share   ☁ Add to Shortcuts   ☆ Favourites   ⏲ Timeout

FRIDAY

⌂ Home   ♡ Share   ☁ Add to Shortcuts   ☆ Favourites   ⏱ Timeout

SATURDAY

⌂ Home   ♡ Share   ☁ Add to Shortcuts   ☆ Favourites   ⏱ Timeout

SUNDAY

Home   ♡ Share   ☁ Add to Shortcuts   ☆ Favourites   ⏱ Timeout

NOTES: A WEEK OF REFLECTIONS

MONDAY

🏠 Home　　♡ Share　　☁ Add to Shortcuts　　☆ Favourites　　⏰ Timeout

TUESDAY

🏠 Home　　♡ Share　　☁ Add to Shortcuts　　☆ Favourites　　⏰ Timeout

WEDNESDAY

⌂ Home ♡ Share ☁ Add to Shortcuts ☆ Favourites ⏰ Timeout

THURSDAY

⌂ Home ♡ Share ☁ Add to Shortcuts ☆ Favourites ⏰ Timeout

FRIDAY

Home   ♡ Share   ☁ Add to Shortcuts   ☆ Favourites   ⏱ Timeout

SATURDAY

Home   ♡ Share   ☁ Add to Shortcuts   ☆ Favourites   ⏱ Timeout

SUNDAY

....

....

....

....

....

....

....

🏠 Home   ♡ Share   ☁ Add to Shortcuts   ☆ Favourites   ⏲ Timeout

NOTES: A WEEK OF REFLECTIONS

....

....

....

....

....

....

....

....

....

....

MONDAY

⌂ Home　　♡ Share　　☁ Add to Shortcuts　　☆ Favourites　　⏱ Timeout

TUESDAY

⌂ Home　　♡ Share　　☁ Add to Shortcuts　　☆ Favourites　　⏱ Timeout

WEDNESDAY

⌂ Home   ♡ Share   ☁ Add to Shortcuts   ☆ Favourites   ⏰ Timeout

THURSDAY

⌂ Home   ♡ Share   ☁ Add to Shortcuts   ☆ Favourites   ⏰ Timeout

FRIDAY

🏠 Home   ♡ Share   ☁ Add to Shortcuts   ☆ Favourites   ⏰ Timeout

SATURDAY

🏠 Home   ♡ Share   ☁ Add to Shortcuts   ☆ Favourites   ⏰ Timeout

SUNDAY

....
....
....
....
....
....
....
....
....

🏠 Home   ♡ Share   ☁ Add to Shortcuts   ☆ Favourites   ⏰ Timeout

NOTES: A WEEK OF REFLECTIONS

....
....
....
....
....
....
....
....
....
....
....

REFERENCES

Chapter 1

1) Lauren, Natural Therapies Practitioner, *Lunaception: Benefits of Aligning Your Cycles with the Moon,* www.empoweredsustenance.com/balance-hormones-with-moon/

2) James J. McKenna et al, ACTA *Paediatrica: An International Journal of Paediatrics,* www.cosleeping.nd.edu/assets/32947/sleep_arousal_synchrony_and_independence_1994.pdf

3) Sian Griffiths, *Co-sleeping Does A Child Good, Peaceful Parenting,* www.drmomma.org/2009/07/co-sleeping-children-should-sleep-with.html

4) USGS Water Science School, *How Much Water Is There On, In, and Above the Earth?,* www.water.usgs.gov/edu/earthhowmuch.html

5) Emarketer, *Smartphone Users Worldwide Will Total 1.75 Billion in 2014,* www.emarketer.com/Article/Smartphone-Users-Worldwide-Will-Total-175-Billion-2014/1010536

Chapter 2

1) Stephanie Watson, Harvard Women's Health Watch, *Volunteering May Be Good for Body and Mind,* www.health.harvard.edu/blog/volunteering-may-be-good-for-body-and-mind-201306266428

2) Kurzweil Accelerating Intelligence, *Walking in Nature Lowers Risk of Depression Scientists Find in MRI Study,* www.kurzweilai.net/walking-in-nature-lowers-risk-of-depression-scientists-find-in-mri-study

3) Nyr Natural News, *Nature is the Best Prescription for Stressed City Dwellers,* www.nyrnaturalnews.com/nature/2015/08/nature-is-the-best-prescription-for-stressed-city-dwellers/

4) Rob Jordan, Stanford Woods Institute for the Environment, *Stanford Researchers Find Mental Health Prescription: Nature,* www.news.stanford.edu/news/2015/june/hiking-mental-health-063015.html

5) David Hershey, MadSci Network, *Water Percentage in Plants,* www.madsci.org/posts/archives/2002-12/1040350077.Bt.r.html

6) Daisy Whitbread, Healthaliciousness.com, *27 Vegetables Highest in Protein,* www.healthaliciousness.com/articles/vegetables-high-in-protein.php

Chapter 3

1) Leah Binder, Forbes.com, *Stunning News On Preventable Deaths In Hospitals,* www.forbes.com/sites/leahbinder/2013/09/23/stunning-news-on-preventable-deaths-in-hospitals/

2) DailyMail.co.uk, *How Stress Can Lead to Stomach Ulcers,* www.dailymail.co.uk/health/article-37953/How-stress-lead-stomach-ulcers.html

3) Sipser, W Dr and Lew, A. (2008) *7 Things Your Doctor Forgot to Tell You,* 3rd Edition, Australia, Rockpool Publishing.

4) TheWaterExpress.com, *Water Facts and Tips,* www.thewaterexpress.com/Water-Facts-And-Tips.htm

Chapter 4

1) Williamson, M. (1996) *A Return to Love: Reflections on the Principles of "A Course in Miracles",* HarperOne.

2) Jack Canfield, *How to Create an Empowering Vision Board,* www. jackcanfield.com/how-to-create-an-empowering-vision-book.

3) Deepak Chopra, M.D. and Rudolph Tanzi, Ph.D., *You Can Transform Your Own Biology,* www.chopra.com/ccl/you-can-transform-your-own-biology

SHOPPING DIRECTORY

Hands On Journeys
www.handsonjourneys.com
Travel with a purpose & give back.

Cocofrio Ice Cream
www.cocofrio.com
Email: yum@cocofrio.com.au

PowerSuperfoods
www.powersuperfoods.com.au

Spiral Foods
www.spiralfoods.com.au

Jomeis Fine Foods
1300 729 626
www.jomeisfinefoods.com.au
Email: info@jomeisfnefoods.com.au

Zazen Alkalized Water
www.zazen.com.au

Generosity Water Australia
www.generositywateraustralia.com
Email: hello@generositywater.com.au

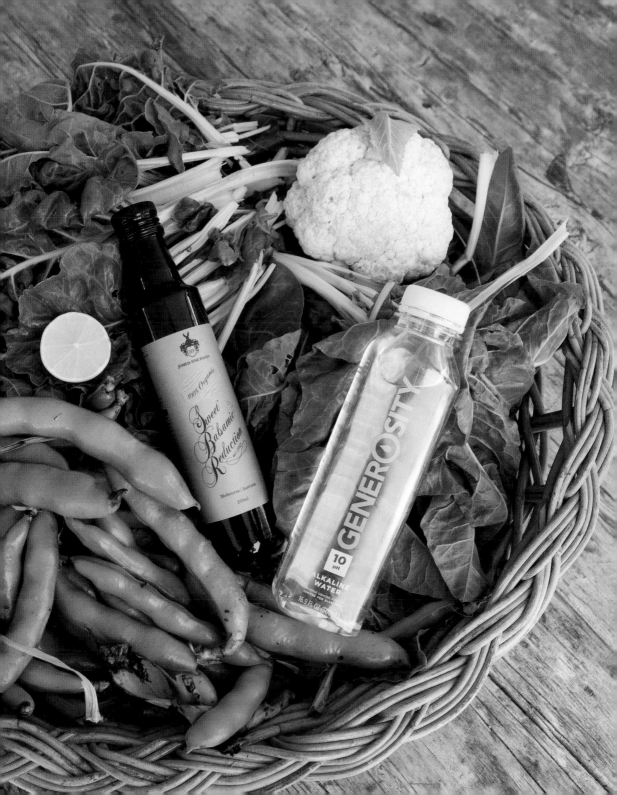

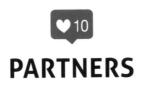

PARTNERS

COCOFRIO Combine a zest for life and health with a love of wholesome food and flavours with Cocofrio, our partner in wellness.

Launched in 2013, Cocofrio had a vision to offer good food and an alternative for lovers of ice-cream that was the healthiest coconut ice-cream in Australia! In less than 12 months, they established themselves as just that, selling their flavourful coconut milk ice-cream Australia-wide with stockists spreading fast.

The company directors Paul and Tintin are passionate producers of food that is good for you. They travel the world sourcing only the best produce. They make sure they listen to customer's needs and change the ingredients to suit the growing trends of consumer's needs.

Cocofrio had a dream of creating an ice-cream that was dairy free and able to be enjoyed as a treat on a daily basis. Because of this, they chose to include only sugar that is plant based and lower GI (Glycemic index). They decided to use no-calorie natural Stevia, creating a dairy, gluten and fructose free ice-cream!

Along with Stevia, Cocofrio ice-cream is also sweetened with organic brown rice malt. Brown rice malt syrup is pure, fructose-free and low GI. It is comprised of 50 percent soluble complex carbohydrates (maltotriose), 45 percent maltose and three percent glucose. Your body digests the maltose in one and a half hours and the complex carbohydrates in three. You absorb the small quantity of glucose immediately. That means a slow and controlled energy release, consistent blood sugar levels, and an even energy flow, with none of the adverse effects other sweeteners can give.

Coconut milk is the key ingredient in Cocofrio ice-cream. It was purposefully chosen to help those with dairy intolerances. Fat from dairy is animal fat, but coconut fat is crammed with medium chain fatty acids, which your body can convert to energy rather than storing as fat. If you do not have the right mix of a healthy, good fat diet and functional fitness movement, animal fats from dairy ice-creams can place you at risk of high cholesterol, arterial flow reduction and coronary disease.

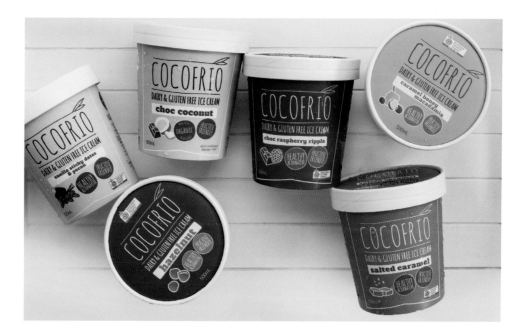

Cocofrio coconut ice-cream also contains omega 6 fatty acids. These are strongly connected to better heart and hormonal health. Other benefits of using coconut include:

Coconut milk is high in lauric acid, one of the active components in human breast milk. It's a key contributor to the formation of a stable immune system, as well as good blood elasticity.
An average serving of coconut milk can provide 22 percent of our daily iron needs.
It contains above average levels of Vitamins C, E, B1, B3, B5, B6 and calcium, magnesium, phosphorus, selenium and sodium. The antioxidant elements also help fight against the free radical process.

Cocofrio is committed to the health of our community so the company has obtained an organic certification from the leading certification agency, ACO (Australian Certification Organic).

Visit **www.cocofrio.com.au** for more information on their products and flavours as well as a wealth of health information and tips. You can find out where to load up your freezer or even how to become a stockist!

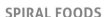

SPIRAL FOODS

Started in the 70's in Melbourne, Australia with a group of alternates, the Spiral Foods company had a desire to follow the Macrobiotic way of life. Since then we have seen many changes in eating patterns and fads but Spiral has maintained its roots.

TODAY.. Spiral Foods is Australia's leading supplier of quality traditional foods with an emphasis on organics. We are now in our fourth decade and our products are found nationally in Australia, New Zealand, South East Asia, Japan, US and Colombia.

Our range includes the finest Organic Oils and Vinegars, traditional foods of Japan, Canadian Maple syrup, Mexican Agave, Organic Fruit Juices and Purees from the US, ready-made organic sauces and drizzles and a large range of local Australian quality groceries.

At Spiral Foods we are proud of our contributions to help slow the unnecessary changes that are occurring to our earth, climate and oceans. Our products are made by people with a passion for wholesome traditional foods of the highest standards and quality.

Good, safe, wholesome food is a basic human right. Our foods continue to provide nourishment and wellbeing across the generations of people who take care about the food they eat and our earth.

We believe good safe wholesome food is a basic human right.

this earth, this food . . .

Visit **www.spiralfoods.com.au** for more information on our products.